THE
GREAT PROSTATE
HOAX

THE
GREAT PROSTATE
HOAX

HOW BIG MEDICINE HIJACKED THE PSA TEST
AND CAUSED A PUBLIC HEALTH DISASTER

RICHARD J. ABLIN, PhD

WITH RONALD PIANA

palgrave
macmillan

First published in 2014 by PALGRAVE MACMILLAN® in the United States—a division of St. Martin's Press LLC, 175 Fifth Avenue, New York, NY 10010.

Where this book is distributed in the UK, Europe, and the rest of the world, this is by Palgrave Macmillan, a division of Macmillan Publishers Limited, registered in England, company number 785998, of Houndmills, Basingstoke, Hampshire RG21 6XS.

Palgrave Macmillan is the global academic imprint of the above companies and has companies and representatives throughout the world.

Palgrave® and Macmillan® are registered trademarks in the United States, the United Kingdom, Europe and other countries.

ISBN 978-1-137-27874-6

Library of Congress Cataloging-in-Publication Data

Ablin, Richard J., 1940– author.
   The great prostate hoax : how big medicine hijacked the PSA test and caused a public health disaster / by Richard J. Ablin, with Ronald Piana.
   p. ; cm.
   Includes bibliographical references.
   ISBN 978-1-137-27874-6 (alk. paper)
   I. Piana, Ron, author. II. Title.
   [DNLM: 1. Prostate-Specific Antigen—adverse effects—United States. 2. Prostatic Neoplasms—diagnosis—United States. 3. Early Detection of Cancer—adverse effects—United States. 4. History, 20th Century—United States. 5. History, 21st Century—United States. 6. Prostate-Specific Antigen—history—United States. WJ 762]
   RC280.P7
   362.19699'463—dc23

                                                    2013030332

A catalogue record of the book is available from the British Library.

Design by Letra Libre, Inc.

First edition: March 2014

10 9 8 7 6 5 4 3 2 1

Printed in the United States of America.

*For the countless millions of men
and their families who have
suffered needlessly because of
the misuse of the PSA Test*

CONTENTS

ACKNOWLEDGMENTS

In the course of writing this book, I have often reflected on the years and events that have passed since I first began my research on the prostate in 1968. Books such as this are built with the help, in one way or another, of numerous people. My wife, Linda, who has been my sounding board for 50 years, warned me not to name names in the likelihood that someone will be overlooked. Nonetheless, it's a risk I need to take. However, if I have omitted you, please understand it was unintentional.

Initially, I must acknowledge the late Ward A. Soanes, MD, who provided me with the wherewithal to pursue my early investigative studies of the prostate. Some years later, 25 in fact, I met Fred Lee, MD, who on introducing me to the late William Cooner, MD, said, "Bill, this is the guy who discovered prostate-specific antigen [PSA]. . . ." Together with the support of Hope T. M. Ritter Jr., PhD (my graduate school professor), Phil Gold, MD, PhD, and the late Lloyd J. Ney Sr., PhD (founder of Patient Advocates for Advanced Cancer Treatments), my discovery of PSA in 1970 was brought to the attention of the biomedical community. Through the intervening years, Eugene V. Genovesi, PhD, Phil Gold, MD, PhD, Mark R. Haythorn, MS, the late John Marchalonis, PhD, Samuel Schluter, PhD, and Terry C. Whyard, MA, have also served as sounding boards for innumerable discussions on PSA. Haythorn, in addition, has been an invaluable resource in keeping me abreast of pertinent biomedical literature. Suzanne B. Connolly, BS, has played a vital role in the preparation of countless audiovisual presentations on my research. And, for those who find this book a compelling and informed read, you owe a debt of gratitude to my son, Michael, who for 17 years has relentlessly urged me to get out the "truth" on the ongoing health care disaster. To accomplish this task, I was most fortunate to have the writing expertise of Ronald Piana. I would also like to acknowledge my colleagues at the University of Arizona College of Medicine and all the interviewees listed in the Appendix. Last, but certainly not least, I wish to thank Karen A. Wolny, Editorial Director at Palgrave Macmillan and her staff for their skilled guidance in publishing this book and finally getting the "truth" out.

Richard J. Ablin, PhD

INTRODUCTION

He's the best physician that knows the worthlessness of most medicines.

—Benjamin Franklin

I wrote this book, in part, as an apology to a man I've never met. Let's call him John, a robust 51-year-old living on a tree-lined street with his wife and kids. He was secretly enjoying the roller-coaster ride of a midlife crisis—a new Corvette, adventurous love-making, ice climbing in New Zealand. Then it happened. During John's yearly physical, his blood work revealed a slightly elevated level of prostate-specific antigen (PSA),[1] an arbitrary indicator of an abnormality in the prostate gland. (The prostate is a gland whose main function is to secrete an alkaline fluid that is an important part of the semen that carries sperm.) After a few clichéd remarks about guideline recommendations, John's primary care physician sent him to a urologist—the doctor-to-doctor handoff that can inadvertently turn men into unwitting victims of a system that may do more harm than good. Why did John enter that system without understanding the life-changing consequences? And how did the misuse of a simple blood test become the engine for a multibillion-dollar industry?

These are some of the questions that I seek to answer. Also, while I was writing this book, several influential organizations, notably the American Urological Association (AUA),[2] adopted more moderate recommendations for PSA screening. This would seem like a good thing. However, in my view it's a case of too little and far too late.

> The PSA blood test is used:
>
> 1. to aid doctors in treating men who already have prostate cancer and to identify the recurrence of prostate cancer following treatment, and
> 2. as a screening test in healthy men to help detect prostate cancer.
>
> This book concerns the misuse of the PSA test for screening healthy men.

For more than 25 years I have publicly denounced mass PSA screening as a public health disaster, most recently in an op-ed piece in the *New York Times* in March 2010.[3] Given my intimate knowledge of the prostate industry, I'm not confident that this medical détente by the AUA will have a significant effect on the continued misuse of PSA. There are dozens of new-generation PSA tests currently being developed, which is simply a more techy way to keep the prostate business rolling full steam ahead. But you can't wash your hands of 30 years of guilt and walk away. This book will also hold those responsible for this human calamity accountable.

Back to John.

Despite the fact that John had no family history of prostate cancer, the urologist advised a better-safe-than-sorry approach and scheduled John for a biopsy. Under local anesthesia, multiple 18-gauge needles were inserted through the skin between his scrotum and rectum and into his prostate gland, punching out core tissue samples. Aside from significant discomfort, this "routine" procedure can hospitalize men with serious infections and bleeding. Although nervous, John and his wife remained cautiously optimistic as they waited for the pathology report. John's mind, however, went on autopilot, plumbing the dark sectors of worst-case scenarios.

When the urologist finally called, the dreaded word *cancer* jolted John into a mind-numbing world of prognosis, extent of cancer, and therapeutic options. The urologist's voice became decidedly upbeat as he informed John that the cancer was confined to the prostate gland. This was good news. Like most prostate cancers, it was probably a "turtle," not a "rabbit" (we'll get to that later in the book). But John was only 51. He wanted the best possible shot at another 30 years; after all, he had plans. His wife panicked as the urologist droned on and on with buoyant pronouncements about survival data and better surgical techniques. At one point, she clasped her husband's hand and blurted, "Cut it out. We want the cancer *gone*." John emphatically agreed.

Like many men in his position, John was caught in the reason-free limbo zone that walled him off from critical thinking. Without searching deeper into the serious clinical implications, he formed his decision in a flash of fear and agreed to a radical prostatectomy—surgery to remove the prostate gland—the suggested option for younger men with localized prostate cancer and a long life expectancy. The surgeon explained the postprocedure complications; most troubling were incontinence and impotence. But the clinical elephant in the room was John's life; it was in the balance, so making the decision to go ahead with surgery was a no-brainer. Why wait?

THERE WAS NO QUESTION that John had prostate cancer, a disease that kills almost 30,000 American men every year. However, most localized cancers never leave the prostate gland and men that have them usually die of other causes, like old age. But important questions were left unasked. For instance, why, at this critical juncture, did the doctor not pause and discuss other viable options such as active surveillance (closely following a patient's condition but not giving treatment unless there are changes in test results; active surveillance may avoid or at least delay the need for treatment). The answer is that doctors, especially urological surgeons, don't get paid to pause. They get paid to prescribe drugs, deliver treatments, and cut. The paradox of harm done by healers with scalpels will feature prominently in a following chapter.

According to the urologist, the operation was a success. John's wife cried happy tears upon hearing that the cancer was gone. But unbeknownst to her at the time, other parts of John were gone also, parts that made John, John. There was postsurgery incontinence, a constant dripping of urine that forced John to wear an absorbent pad—his diaper, as he wryly called it. Worse, the surgery had left him impotent—a year after being "cured," John still couldn't have sex with his wife.

The clinical explanation for John's impotence—temporary cavernous nerve damage (neuropraxia) resulting in penile hypoxia, smooth muscle apoptosis, fibrosis, and venoocclusive dysfunction—offered no solace to the emptiness in his marriage. Neither did the many erectile dysfunction drugs or the follow-up visits with one doctor after another. John simply wasn't the man he used to be and doubted that he ever would be. This left him wondering if the rest of his life would unfold in the captivity of impotence and self-doubt. And what about the damage to his marriage?

SO WHY DO I FEEL THE NEED to apologize to John, the everyman of prostate cancer whom I've never met? Although complicated, the answer begins with a simple fact: I discovered PSA in 1970.[4] And by virtue of that scientific find, I have been linked to the 30 million American men, like John, who undergo routine PSA screening for prostate cancer. The result: a million needle biopsies per year, leading to more than 100,000 radical prostatectomies, *most of which are unnecessary.*

One thing that crystalizes many of the daunting questions in this health care story is our national, almost religious, predilection to believe in *tests* themselves. We generally agree that routine cholesterol testing decreases heart disease, targeted mammography screening reduces breast cancer mortality, and timely colon-cancer tests ultimately save lives. So, on the surface, PSA testing sounds like another good way to catch disease early, when it is most curable. Naturally, with our health at stake, we have a universal desire to hear the word "normal" attached to a test result. Therein lies the rub; there is no *normal* when it comes to PSA.

Down to basics: PSA is a protein (proteins are fundamental components of all living cells and include many substances, such as enzymes, hormones, and antibodies, which are necessary for the proper functioning of an organism) whose chief duty is to liquefy ejaculated semen, allowing sperm cells to swim freely on their exquisitely challenged mission—conceiving human life. The PSA test measures the amount of PSA that's released by the prostate gland into the blood. However, since the majority of PSA is carried in the semen, the technology only gauges the minute amount that escapes into the blood stream. To grasp the minuteness we're talking about, PSA is measured in billionths of a gram per thousandths of a liter (ng/mL)!

Aside from our national devotion to tests, we're also fixated on numbers. The PSA number currently used as the highest *normal* level is 4 ng/mL. A well-known urologist, who you'll meet later, argued passionately that the number for recommending needle biopsy should be reduced to 2.5 ng/mL, which would markedly increase the amount of biopsies performed on men, most of which would end up as benign. It is vital to understand that a man might have a PSA of 0.5 and have prostate cancer, yet another man whose number is an alarming 11 could be cancer free. In a following chapter, I'll drill deeper into the numbers and how they should be used in the context of prostate health.

Further complicating the matter of interpreting the numbers, PSA levels are affected by a host of factors *un*related to cancer. For example, if a long-haul truck driver barreling over the Grand Tetons at night stops in a clinic the next morning to have a blood test, the jostling ride over the mountains could have elevated his PSA level. An amorous motel romp that evening could further elevate the level. So might a relatively common condition known as benign prostatic hyperplasia (BPH) (enlarged prostate) or another condition known as prostatitis (inflammation of the prostate). The list of possible offenders goes on, but the outcome of PSA testing remains the same: the level is affected by numerous stimuli and the numbers do not necessarily indicate cancer.

So, for the past several decades—in the scientific and public forum, from Arizona, where I live and work, to far-flung places such as Kolkata (Calcutta), India where I was received by Mother Teresa, and medical conferences in Dar es Salaam, Tanzania—I have been stating unequivocally that PSA is simply a normal component of the prostate. It is *not* specific for cancer. Rather, it is present in the normal, benign, *and* cancerous prostate. I did not call PSA "prostate *cancer*-specific antigen" because it is not an indicator that prostate cancer exists. The PSA test is therefore not an appropriate tool for early diagnosis of prostate cancer, as some of the self-anointed experts continue to stubbornly preach. Put simply, the ability of the PSA test to identify men with prostate cancer is slightly better than that of flipping a coin. And its continued use as a routine screening tool is nothing short of a national health disaster.

THE ROOTS OF THIS STORY reach back to the dawn of scientific inquiry, when men first began offering theories about the unknown. As the scientist who discovered PSA, I confess to an elite thrill that my ilk shares; looking into a microscope is like peering into the unknown reaches of space, trying to see something that no one before you has seen. But for all the groundbreaking discoveries that have bettered humankind, science is also a double-edged sword, bookended by greed and ego.

Unabashed greed was on public display when US tobacco companies joined forces and deliberately confused the debate about smoking and cancer by creating and funding "scientific" research organizations that never intended to connect tobacco with lung malignancies. Even after the surgeon general's 1964 report *Smoking and Health* left no doubt about the insidious connection between cigarettes and lung cancer, Big Tobacco referenced qualified scientists who challenged that evidence. In short, it was science for sale and, almost a half-century later, lung cancer remains the number one cause of cancer death in the United States.

Several decades later, between 1990 and 1995, we saw the results of an unfettered scientific ego. Werner Bezwoda, MD, PhD, a doctor in Johannesburg, South Africa, led numerous clinical studies of a breakthrough treatment for high-risk breast-cancer patients. The treatment—high-dose chemotherapy with bone marrow transplantation—cost $100,000 and had brutal side effects. But these women were desperate for a cure, and after a groundswell of emotional advocacy the treatment was approved; 30,000 American women subsequently underwent this physically debilitating ordeal only to find out that Bezwoda had falsified the results of his studies in his doomed quest for fame.[5] His supersized ego had warped the ethical foundation doctors are supposed to live by, leaving 30,000 hopelessly damaged women in its wake.

To fully comprehend this type of science for sale, whether for pure monetary gain or boundless ego or, as I point out in this book, *both*, one must first understand that it's a nuanced tale ranging from out-and-out deceit to subliminally formed, wrong-headed decisions. For instance, in 1994, with questionable supporting evidence and without considering the possible benefit versus harm to men, the US Food and Drug Administration (FDA) made a fateful error and approved PSA testing as a means to *detect* prostate cancer, opening the floodgates for a tsunami of routine nationwide testing. A doctor you'll meet later, Stanford University urologist Thomas A. Stamey, MD, was an early and aggressive proponent of PSA testing. He later recanted his soapbox advocacy for the test, lamenting that most of the prostatectomies performed at Stanford hospital were unnecessary.[6] Dr. Stamey's late-career mea culpa over egregious patterns of needless surgeries leads to the larger question: *How did this gross misuse of science happen?*

To answer that question, I'll delve deeply into the truly astonishing discrepancies between prostate cancer fact and fiction and the billion-dollar lies told about the detection of this disease. But in a larger sense, the situation dramatized by John illustrates the grim reality of the health care system itself: encouraged by perverse incentives, many of the tests and procedures that doctors do are unnecessary, and quite a few are downright harmful. For example, in studies stretching from the mid-1980s to the late 1990s, RAND Health[7] researchers found that up to one-third of selected medical procedures were performed for inappropriate reasons and had questionable benefits. That sad finding is the result, in part, of a payment system that financially encourages doctors to overtreat patients, despite knowing that overtreatment is blatant malpractice with serious medical consequences. I revisit this theme in the pages that follow.

As I've mentioned, health, science, and medicine cannot be fully separated from greed and ego. Big money lubricates the prostate cancer machine and I'll explore the belly of that beast throughout this book. But this is a story about men and women deeply hurt by those they trusted. In today's vernacular, primary care doctors, like the one who sent John to the urologist, are termed gatekeepers, because they open the portals to specialists and the medical trail ahead. But the system itself should be a gatekeeper. The FDA, for instance, is the main gatekeeper charged with ensuring the drugs and medical devices that go into the market, such as the PSA test, are not only safe but that they adhere to the most important principle in medicine: *First, do no harm*. Most Americans know more about the internal workings of their cars than they do about their bodies. We trust our doctors to prevent illness and cure it if it strikes. At the very least, we expect that they do no harm.

I am a professor of pathology at the University of Arizona College of Medicine, the Arizona Cancer Center, and BIO5 Institute. In 1979, in memory of my father, I founded the Robert Benjamin Ablin Foundation for Cancer Research. I, along with others, am still searching for a true prostate *cancer*-specific marker. It is my aim with this book to shed light on the devastating human consequences of manipulating science for personal and financial gain and to raise provocative questions about the very nature of our health care system, hopefully fostering positive change in the process.

ONE

THE JUNGLE

Great doubt: great awakening.
Little doubt: little awakening.
No doubt: no awakening.

—Zen Maxim

Power is the ultimate aphrodisiac.

—Henry Kissinger

It would come to me several years after I discovered PSA, an internal stirring that something I was part of was going terribly wrong. A scientific sleight of hand had recklessly sparked a destructive wildfire of false hope in our health system—I knew it would be near impossible to confine, let alone put out. If it had but one name I'd call it *potestas*, Latin for power. Money usually plays a leading role in abuse-of-power stories. It does in the one you are about to read.

I never imagined how society's collective mind could be warped by fear until my days as a US Agency for International Development Research Consultant in Asuncion, Paraguay. I was there investigating better ways to diagnose and treat Chagas disease,[1] which is caused by the protozoan *Trypanosoma cruzi* and vectored to humans by the parasitic "kissing bug," *Triatoma*. My work took me from a laboratory at the University of Asuncion out to sun-scorched rural areas where locals guided me through mud-hut villages festering with *Triatoma*.

At that time, Paraguay was clenched in the iron grip of the military dictator Alfredo Stroessner. My associates at the lab confided that Stroessner, paranoid about a leftist coup d'état, had his thugs spirit away suspected communists, shoving them out of airplanes soaring thousands of feet above the obliterating jungle.

Monsters like Stroessner won't appear again in this story. But you will meet powerful men in white lab coats who manipulated our medical system for personal gain and self-aggrandizement, setting in motion a self-perpetuating industry that has maimed millions of American men—and continues to do so.

Our scientific and medical history tells us, among other things, that actions based on contrived evidence and the people behind those actions can grow old together unless exposed with a loud enough voice. The word science is derived from the Latin *scientia,* meaning *knowledge*. What good is knowledge without evidence?

DISCOVERY

After finishing my work in Paraguay, I returned to the States and completed my US Postdoctoral Fellowship in the internationally renowned Bacteriology and Immunology Department at the University of Buffalo School of Medicine. It was 1968, a fiery year—the Vietnam War was still raging, Martin Luther King Jr. was gunned down at a motel in Memphis, igniting nationwide riots, and Richard Nixon's obsession with winning the presidency was consummated. Challenging social norms was the zeitgeist of the late sixties and for a young immunologist consumed with investigating the hidden structure and function of cells there has never been a freewheeling time like it.

Scientific research is a rigidly disciplined process, but serendipity has long played a role in notable careers and discoveries, as it did in mine. In short, my postdoctoral mentor traded me to the Millard Fillmore Hospital Research Institute (an affiliate of the University of

Buffalo School of Medicine), for a fluorescent microscope he needed for his own lab. The gist of the deal was, "Give me a fluorescent microscope and you can have Ablin." Of course, the details of that swap were more complicated, shrouded in academic intrigue that I won't retrace. After the microscope was delivered, I joined the institute and worked with two urologists, Drs. Ward A. Soanes and Maurice J. Gonder. As it turned out, Soanes and Gonder had a generous grant from the John A. Hartford Foundation funding their studies of the normal and abnormal prostate gland. Being traded for a microscope worked out just fine.

Soanes, who co-owned several private hospitals, was a snazzy dresser who tooled around the city of Buffalo in a Rolls-Royce Silver Shadow. His more conservative counterpart, Gonder, was a square-jawed man with a military bearing. Cosmetic differences aside, the two urologists had developed cryosurgery—now known as cryoablation[2]—and were investigating its then novel role in prostate cancer, which I found a captivating line of scientific inquiry.

At first we experimented with cryosurgery on the prostate of rabbits and rhesus monkeys, in which we observed an interesting immune response. As the research progressed, we began treating the prostate of cancer patients with cryosurgery; several men had advanced disease that had spread to distant areas such as the lungs and cervical vertebrae. Following their cryosurgery, I witnessed a spellbinding phenomenon—distant tumors had regressed; in some cases all of the patient's cancer had *vanished*.[3]

Naturally, I wanted to know how freezing the primary tumor enacted such an explosive immune response, for which I coined the term *cryoimmunotherapy*.[4] I went seeking an answer. The lab animals we treated with cryotherapy had an immune response to antigens[5] of the frozen tumor tissue. Since I saw similar responses in men with prostate cancer, I hypothesized as one possible explanation that the frozen-tissue destruction might have liberated a prostate cancer-specific antigen responsible for the cryoimmunotherapeutic effect.[6]

Sensing a breakthrough, I immediately launched a series of immunologic studies of the normal, benign, and malignant human prostate and secretions to determine whether a cancer-specific anti-gen was at work. I could not find one (I, along with others, am still looking), but I did discover a prostate tissue-specific antigen—PSA. The year was 1970.[7]

THE "DOCTOR" DOTH PROTEST TOO MUCH, METHINKS

In 1953 two scientists, James Watson and Francis Crick, sauntered into the Eagle Pub in Cambridge, England, and announced they had found *the secret of life:* DNA. From antiquity until the present, sci-entific discovery in many instances has always been a messy affair of unrequited recognition. Not surprising, a nasty dispute over Watson and Crick's discovery still surfaces in the national press every so of-ten. I didn't discover the secret of life, but my discovery of PSA as a biomarker is noted as a major scientific advance. As with DNA, PSA has not been immune to controversy. For several decades, a coterie of powerful doctors has tried to discredit my discovery. Since their compulsion to silence my message about PSA screening is a core ele-ment of this book, I'll clear the issue up before moving on.

I left Buffalo in mid-1970, moving with my wife, Linda, our son, Michael, and our Irish Setter, Deacon, to Springfield, Illinois. There, I headed up the immunological component of a developing renal trans-plant program at Memorial Hospital of Springfield in affiliation with the Southern Illinois University School of Medicine. In early 1973, on the invitation of two urologists at Chicago's Cook County Hospital, I had the opportunity to return to my research on the prostate and we all moved to Chicago, where I began a ten-year stint at Cook County Hospital and the Hektoen Institute for Medical Research.

Nothing notable happened in the PSA story until 1979, when a group from Roswell Park Cancer Institute (RPCI, located in Buffalo, New York)[8] published a paper in the journal *Investigative Urology* claiming the discovery of PSA.[9] One of the paper's authors, T. Ming Chu, contended that his PSA was different from mine. It doesn't serve this book's purpose to delve into dense scientific analysis over the an-tigens, but for clarity it is important for the reader to understand that

PSA, no matter who discovered it, is not *cancer*-specific—therefore it cannot not detect prostate cancer. That is a critical point to grasp as we move forward, because it is the lynchpin of my argument against using PSA to screen healthy men for prostate cancer. In chapter 3, I'll make my position clear, using a set of easy-to-understand principles I call the *four cruxes*.

The dispute with Roswell Park has been publicly debated in letters to the editor and commentaries across multiple journals, which ultimately proved nothing, settling like windblown ashes on a cold fire.[10] Today the firm consensus among the scientific community is: in 1970 Ablin initially observed PSA; in 1979 Roswell Park's Chu and other researchers set out to extend Ablin's initial discovery by purifying and characterizing[11] PSA and subsequently developing the PSA test.[12]

I have never challenged that narrative, only the misuse of the molecule that I discovered.

In 1984 Roswell Park received a patent for an immunoassay blood test in prostate cancer. The technology was transferred to the biomedical industry, a clumsy handoff during which the nuanced benefits of PSA (discussed in later chapters) were cleverly distorted into a prostate cancer-screening tool and mass marketed to eager but uninformed doctors and their patients. In Chu's own words, "Things started happening quickly after that."[13] They certainly did. In the next chapter I'll flash forward two years to a critical juncture and explore how the clinical truth of the PSA test was either manipulated and or disregarded by the biotech industry, the US government, and the urology community.

A bit about Roswell Park Cancer Institute. It is difficult for the lay reader to comprehend the embedded power in an institution such as Roswell Park. Its designation as the first National Cancer Institute (NCI) Comprehensive Cancer Center distinguishes Roswell as a crown jewel in our $3 trillion-per-year health care system. For decades, doctors in this powerful bully pulpit have consistently silenced, by dint of their authority, any challenge to their dogma on PSA screening. For example, in September 2012 Roswell's president and CEO, Donald L. Trump, MD, and its chair of urology, James Mohler, MD, using the age-old practice of casting doubt on the messenger to cast doubt on the message, wrote a tortuous, condescending letter to the editor of *The ASCO Post* in an attempt to discredit my discovery of PSA.[14]

More disturbing is their use of the unjustified fear of cancer as some kind of human shield to protect their position, stating that my and the US Preventive Services Task Force's[15] strong recommendation against PSA screening in asymptomatic men would "certainly return us to the days when most men . . . were likely to die a long, painful death from [prostate cancer]."

Although the moat protecting the PSA fortress is beginning to dry up, its defenders still man the parapets. Otis Brawley, MD, a prominent oncologist who is the chief medical officer of the American Cancer Society, was once a proponent of routine PSA screening. But over the past several years, Brawley has modified his view, becoming skeptical of tactics used to push mass routine PSA screening, saying that he's "against lying to men . . . exaggerating the evidence to get men screened."[16] To Brawley's heresy Mohler responded, "I have known Otis for over 20 years. He doesn't come off as being ignorant or stupid, but when it comes to prostate-cancer screening he must not be as intelligent as he seems."[17] It is worth noting that Mohler, who is very high up on the political food chain in the health care industry, chooses his words with care.

Trump and Mohler, and others you'll soon meet, may continue their efforts to discredit my role in the PSA saga and challenge others who share my opinion. But my message is based on science, not self-serving rancor: routine PSA screening does far more harm to men than good and the potential harms can be crippling and life-changing.

WAR

As Susan Sontag wrote in her classic work *Illness as Metaphor,* "The controlling metaphors in the descriptions of cancer are, in fact . . .

drawn from the language of warfare."[18] We officially began our war in 1971, when Richard Nixon signed the National Cancer Act, which was the opening salvo in the so-called War on Cancer. Waging war gave the people an enemy, something to rally around. Jingoism might have its place in actual war, but *not* in medicine—evidence should always trump emotion. A gold-rush mentality to embrace the next greatest medical breakthrough can, as in the PSA test, have dire consequences.

The timing for mass marketing was perfect. Promising studies in breast mammography fueled a national explosion of cancer screening. The feminist movement brought discussion of breast cancer out of the closet. Advocacy groups, led by formidable women, lobbied on Capitol Hill for universal breast cancer screening. The mantra "early detection leads to cure," chanted by breast cancer advocates, would soon be embedded in our national consciousness. By the early 1980s men had grown restless for their own early detection tool. Prostate cancer had a visceral grip on men akin to that of breast cancer on women; it spoke directly to gender-based fear of premature mortality and struck at the core of manhood. Men would begin to form their own advocacy groups, using celebrity prostate cancer survivors as spokesmen.

As the screening storm kicked up, the emerging biotech industry and the urology community focused their collective energies on an irresistible financial opportunity: 30 million age-appropriate American men. The word *campaign*—with its militaristic connotation of confronting an enemy—was rolled out like tanks by the marketing machines that ginned up the prostate cancer business model. Stakeholders from major cancer organizations to the federal government— for example, in 1999 the Postal Service issued a stamp advocating annual PSA tests—tacitly urged on the campaign by turning a blind eye to an uncomfortable scientific fact: I tried to explain that PSA does not detect prostate cancer simply because it is not a cancer-specific marker. Even its most ardent proponents don't challenge that scientific fact. In pages to come, I'll break the PSA test down to its constituent parts and illustrate the downstream clinical effects its routine misuse has on men and the unvarnished human realities of unnecessary procedures.

To illustrate a critical theme of this book, I'll tip my hat to Sontag's war metaphor. Doctors need tools to diagnose illness. Patients wait nervously for the results of the diagnostic tests their doctors order. Unfortunately, our diagnostic technology does not always tell the clinical truth. It can produce a false negative (the test missed detecting something, such as a tumor) or, more likely, and more pertinent to this story, a false positive (indicating a condition that does not exist, such as cancer).

In 2003, while the country was still cocooned in post-9/11 fear, the United States made war on Iraq. History will judge that aggression. However, using the war as a medical metaphor serves this story well. In making the case to the American people, the Bush administration and the lay press referred to Saddam Hussein as a *cancer* whose weapons of mass destruction (WMDs) would *metastasize* throughout the region, eventually to our shores. Surveillance planes (think PSA screening) picked up what was roundly purported to be evidence of the vaunted WMDs. Of course there never were any WMDs. The urgent need to wage war was emotionally based on a monumental false positive that was sold to an American public still numb from the catastrophe on 9/11.

The way the PSA test has been misused for more than three decades amounts to the most damaging false positive in American medical history. How could we reiterate a medical blunder for 30 years? When powerful people repeat an idea often enough—even when it is false—a mind-blunting form of authority is established, and getting there can be an alarmingly swift process. Confronting the imbedded medical authority is where the battle over the trust and value of American health care might very well be won or lost.

TWO

A DECISION I THOUGHT
I COULD LIVE WITH

*It is a predisposition of human nature to consider an unpleasant
idea untrue, and then it is easy to find arguments against it.*

—Sigmund Freud

*Has there ever been a society that has died of dissent? Several have
died of conformity in our lifetime.*

—Jacob Bronowski

On a rainy October night in 1979 I was catching up on my
reading when a paper in the journal *Investigative Urology*,
"Purification of a Human Prostate Specific Antigen (PSA),"[1]
caught my attention. I wasn't surprised to see that the authors were
from Roswell Park Cancer Institute. Over the years—despite the
controversy over whether I or Roswell's T. Ming Chu actually discovered PSA—I'd considered Roswell's investigations on the antigen
as a theoretical curiosity, not fully sure of their endpoint. I dwelled
in a simple academic ethos: you make a discovery, you publish a
few journal papers, you move on. However, a follow-up 1980 article
in the journal *Cancer Research* indicated that Roswell had grander
ambitions for the molecule I first observed in 1970.[2]

Although concerned about the grave potential for misusing PSA, at that time I was absorbed with, among other things, my research in immunotherapy at Cook County Hospital in Chicago. But as PSA screening began rolling out across America, I felt as though I were rubbernecking one of those multivehicle disasters in which dense fog sneaks up and blankets a stretch of highway. Cars, one after another, ram into each other, setting off a massive chain reaction crash. The full damage can only be calculated after the weather clears.

The early PSA papers out of Roswell had also caught the attention of some entrepreneurial-minded scientists in San Diego. Still in their 20s and working out of a laboratory cobbled together from trailers, these young scientists were at the cutting edge of the soon-to-boom biotech industry. (In its simplest definition, biotechnology, or biotech is the use of living systems and organisms to develop or make products such as pharmaceutical therapies and diagnostic tests.) Within several years they'd be known in San Diego lore as the "test-tube cowboys" of a white-hot start-up company named Hybritech. Cofounded by Howard Birndof and Ivor Royston, Hybritech quickly became a magnet for talent, drawing postdocs out of the staid "publish-or-perish" world of academia. In less than a decade, amid infringement lawsuits they filed to protect their patent,[3] and takeovers by larger companies, the vernacular of Hybritech would be not only be science, but Wall Street, IPOs, stock options, and terms like *burn rate*. Many of Hybritech's alumni became rich and famous, largely due to their most successful product, the Hybritech Tandem-R PSA assay (test).

It's important to note that Hybritech and other successful fledgling biotech firms in San Diego signaled a cultural transformation in the way drugs and medical devices move from the point of discovery to market and, ultimately, into the doctor-patient setting. This capitalist dreamscape, where science and industry morphed into one entity, foreshadowed the modern medical industry. Today, the private sector's capital spending on research has exceeded spending by the public (government) and academic sectors combined.[4] Of course, money has always been a major incentive for bright people to pursue risky ventures. Bill Gates and Steve Jobs became fabulously wealthy and also bettered our lives with their products. Similarly, scientific advances bankrolled by the private sector are driven largely by money. But there's an important distinction in the principle of supply and demand—you choose to buy a laptop or computer program; you don't choose to become a patient needing medical care. And, for good reasons, the doctor-patient relationship is founded on a time-honored social compact of trust, not a paper warranty glued to the back of a product.

Most health care consumers know little to nothing about how medical products—such as the diagnostic device central to this story—are developed, approved, and marketed to the public, even though their lives depend on it. Over the past few decades, the pharmaceutical industry has wielded immense influence over the regulatory processes that are supposed to weed out ineffective and unsafe products. And in doing so, these drug manufacturing giants have engaged in a willful disconnect from hard scientific evidence in order to exploit the captive health care market. For instance, a recent study[5] by researchers at the University of California San Francisco has found that "papers reporting the results of industry-sponsored studies present a far more favorable picture of the effects of drugs and medical devices than those reporting on studies that were not sponsored by industry."

Previous studies, papers, and books have described this conflict-of-interest culture that is endemic in medical industries. But industry leaders, with deep pockets and powerful connections, regard academic whistleblowers with a removed hauteur as they go about their business. Of course, caricaturizing any entity or industry as a greed-blinded villain bilking the system would be far too facile and overly cynical. There are many scrambled pieces in the narrative that began with my discovery of PSA—now I'll begin arranging those pieces at one of the story's inflection points: Hybritech.

THE PRODUCT

Birndorf and Royston founded Hybritech in 1978 like surfers catching the crest of a huge wave—the wave being the rise of the new monoclonal antibodies technology. This technology formed the backbone of their proposed business model of developing a line of medical diagnostic devices. The invention of hybridoma technology sped the monoclonal antibody process. (A hybridoma cell is a fusion of two other cell types called B-lymphocytes and myeloma cells.) It's not essential to plumb the depths of cellular biology, but briefly describing the technology that fueled Hybritech's success adds context to the larger story of how certain health care products develop their own markets. And, as you'll see, once a product is embraced and promoted in the health system it's very hard for the US Food and Drug Administration (FDA) to monitor its safe use, even when things go wrong.

Our bodies defend themselves with antibodies, which are created by the immune system's ability to target and kill invading organisms. The immune system recognizes foreign molecules, or *antigens,* and sends antibodies to destroy them. Before monoclonal antibodies, if you wanted to make an antibody for a particular type of bacteria, you would inject an animal with the bacteria; the animal's system would produce antibodies to fight the bacteria; you then bled the animal, separated the serum (the liquid part of the blood), and you would have antibodies to use in vaccines, for example.

For the Hybritech scientists, there were two problems: First, within serum there are hundreds of types of antibodies and to develop a diagnostic device, such as the PSA test, they needed to isolate an antibody that could reproduce identical copies of itself—*mono*clonal as opposed to *poly*clonal. Second, to mass-produce a diagnostic test they needed an unlimited supply of a specific antibody, which was not available until 1975, when two Nobel laureates, Cesar Milstein and Georges Kohler, solved those problems by developing the hybridoma technique for the production of monoclonal antibodies. This technique can detect bacterial, viral, or tumor antigens that are present in the smallest amounts of blood. Think of hybridoma technology as a biological machine. It mass-produces identical units called monoclonal antibodies that are attracted to specific antigens in the blood serum and can detect their level. That was Hybritech's goal for the PSA test: to find the certain levels of the antigen in the blood that would be used to diagnose prostate cancer.

Diagnostic tests are the safety nets of medicine; we fully expect lab results to be infallible predictors of our health status. An inward sigh of relief usually follows a doctor's utterance, "The results were negative." Unfortunately, diagnostic tests are subject to an alarming array of factors that can produce incorrect findings. The consequences can be devastating. I'll drill deeper into the troubling vagaries of lab results as they pertain to PSA, most importantly, why the PSA test does not do what it purports to do.

BIRNDORF AND ROYSTON[6] came from similarly humble beginnings. Birndorf, born in 1950, grew up in a working-class Jewish neighborhood in Detroit; his father was a traveling shoe salesman who often left Monday mornings with his shoe samples and did not return until the end of the week. Royston's parents were Eastern European Jews who met in London during the chaos of World War II; his father, a hardscrabble sheet metal worker, moved the family from England to the United States in 1954. The future biotech partners met at Stanford University; Birndorf was a biochemist working as a lab tech and Royston, who already had an MD from Johns Hopkins, was doing an oncology fellowship. Royston envisioned a prestigious academic career, including grandiose dreams of finding a silver-bullet cure for cancer. The actual circumstance of their first meeting depends on who tells the story. Birndorf's version is simple: "Ivor was in the lab putzing around himself and we met. We struck up a friendship."

Monoclonal antibody technology was abuzz in San Diego's scientific community and Royston smelled an opportunity. At the onset, his partnership with Birndorf was uneven. Royston was five years older than Birndorf and he had an MD degree whereas Birndorf had only an MS. Royston, a hyperkinetic go-getter—who had dabbled in finance ventures as early as high school—also had an entrepreneurial edge over Birndorf. An associate summed up the partners' skill sets regarding the budding monoclonal antibody business: "Ivor knew how to talk about them, but Howard knew how to make them."

Royston's ability to "talk about them" attracted Brook Beyers, an associate at the legendary venture capital firm Kleiner-Perkins. After an initial meeting, Beyers brought his firm's founder, Thomas Perkins, into the picture. According to Birndorf, he and Royston met Beyers and Perkins at an airport bar, hammering out a deal on the back of a cocktail napkin, after which Perkins cut a check for $300,000 in seed money. They called the company Hybritech.

Just prior to Hybritech, Perkins had funded another biotech start-up, Genentech, destined to become a giant in the international pharmaceutical industry. Perkins would become Genentech's chairman, one of the crowning achievements in a life of glittering successes. Perkins, whose understated chutzpah symbolized the biotech phenomenon that erupted in the late 1970s, was described by one of his associates, Thomas D. Kiley: "Tom Perkins wears charisma in the easy way a fine Italian suit drapes the shoulders. In his presence you begin to understand the impact President John Fitzgerald Kennedy had on those around him—the world seems morning fresh, bathed in photographer's light. His attention makes you feel special."[7]

At first, Perkins organized and ran Hybritech's corporate affairs, using Genentech as a business template. Past Hybritech employees unanimously chant praises of the company's freewheeling scientific culture; they arrived at work early and left late, including on weekends. A beer keg greeted them each Friday afternoon. Hybritech's unscripted environment, designed for young scientists, was an enticing recruiting tool. Searching for talent, Birndorf approached a restless young PhD named Gary David, who had a reputation as an ultracreative protein chemist. Hybritech was a perfect fit and David was welcomed aboard. He would ultimately serve a key role in Hybritech's R&D program.

This is where the story takes a turn.

The most seductive product in the biotech business is the block-buster cancer drug. The term *blockbuster* is usually earmarked for what's known as a billion-dollar drug. In the music industry it would be the equivalent of a recording that goes platinum. But with enormous revenue potential comes equally enormous risk—the drug development pipeline is littered with costly white elephants that died before reaching FDA review.

By 1981 Hybritech was becoming an industry leader in hybridoma technology. The company's young scientists were recognized as leaders in the emerging field of monoclonal antibodies. The biotech explosion had become a national fascination. Wall Street was teeming with IPOs for companies investigating mysterious cancer drugs with hard-to-pronounce names. Royston had his sights set on building future fortunes in cancer therapeutics, but there was far too much risk for his still-new company. Hybritech needed a safer revenue-generating product. According to Royston, it was CEO Howard E. (Ted) Greene that proposed a plan. "Ted's idea was, 'Let's come up with a diagnostic [test] strategy to bring in near-term revenues, while we build our therapeutics program, because you don't need FDA-approval for that." Of course, you do need FDA approval to sell a diagnostic device. Greene was loosely referencing the comparative ease of getting approval for a diagnostic device as compared with getting approval for a cancer drug.

The pharmaceutical powerhouse Abbott had already staked out a corner of the market with its product, Ausria, a radioimmunoassay test to detect hepatitis. There was no point in going head-to-head with Abbott's hepatitis test. Royston credits their new scientist David with offering an alternative: "I've been reading about this new antigen called PSA, and it was developed, discovered [*sic*] and characterized in Roswell Park and they claimed that it is secreted in patients with prostate cancer and might be a marker for prostate cancer. Why don't we make an antibody for that [PSA] and develop a test for prostate cancer?"

The decision to develop the PSA test seemed so simple, bordering on cavalier: men sitting around a table looking for a product to fill a market. The way Royston relates the story they might as well have been playing cards. Yes, Hybritech was a for-profit business and the decision to launch a new product was filtered through a risk calculation that lives or dies on the balance sheet. What puzzles me is that these men were scientists who inexplicably failed to recognize the fact that PSA is not cancer-specific and cannot serve as a test to detect prostate cancer. Perhaps they were blinded by lavish dreams of using the PSA test as a cash cow to facilitate Hybritech's march into the rarified therapeutics market, where potential blockbuster cancer drugs lurk.

My longtime colleague and friend, Philip Gold, MD, PhD, whose discovery of carcinoembryonic antigen (CEA) in 1965 ushered in the modern era of tumor markers, had a simpler take on Hybritech's convenient PSA myopia. "There's no debate, Richard Ablin discovered PSA. He was always clear that it was not cancer-specific, but those early studies supporting PSA's potential as a predictor of prostate cancer came out of Roswell Park, America's first comprehensive cancer center. That's all the evidence Hybritech needed, so why look further?"[8]

Royston, in his customary reductionist style, said that they licensed the PSA antigen from Roswell Park, "which took forever." With David in the lead, Hybritech's R&D team began developing the Hybritech Tandem-R PSA assay, noting how "once we got it working and testing people's blood and seeing how it correlated . . . we saw positive tests in males before they [were] diagnosed with prostate cancer . . . finding out that we could diagnose it."[9]

Despite the luster of Roswell Park's imprimatur, there was no convincing scientific evidence to support Royston's goal that the test they developed could serve as a diagnostic tool. The main problem with this theory is that PSA is not prostate cancer-specific; in other words, there is no specific number that indicates prostate cancer. I'll explain this in depth in the following chapter.

Everyone in the diagnostics arena wants a test with the predictive power of what is perhaps the most successful screening tool in medicine: the Papanicolaou test, known as the Pap smear. A speculum is used to open the vaginal canal, cells are swabbed from the cervix and examined under a microscope; the cells are identified as normal, precancerous, or cancerous—a simple test that has dramatically reduced cervical cancer deaths. Not so with PSA, and the explanation of why PSA testing does not reduce prostate cancer mortality does not hinge on entirely predictable events.

The PSA test would become the cash cow that Royston and the others had hoped for, but not for Hybritech as they knew it. During the development period, Hybritech's well-known skill in hybridoma technology and monoclonal antibodies had hooked one of the bigger fish in the pharmaceutical waters, Eli Lilly, a global pharmaceutical company that traces its roots back to 1876. Lilly, the first company to mass-produce penicillin, now has operations in about 125 countries.

Lilly's secret overtures to Hybritech began in 1984, culminating with the sale of Hybritech to the global giant on September 18, 1985. The merger made people at Hybritech rich. CEO Greene tried to assure Hybritech's staff that nothing would change. (That wasn't entirely the case; according to one of Hybritech's scientists, as soon as the brass at Eli Lilly saw the beer mug emblem flying on the company flag, it came down.) Before going to market, the Hybritech Tandem-R PSA test had one major hurdle: FDA approval. In a way, the approval process is like a trial and, as you'll see, the jury was mixed. Even so, it was a decision I *thought* I could live with.

BEDPANS TO BRAIN SCANS

During my research for this book, as I began putting together the puzzle of how PSA became the fulcrum of the multibillion-dollar prostate cancer industry, I was drawn to a frank but telling statement by Hybritech moneyman, Tom Perkins. Over his robust venture capitalist career, Perkins had many dealings with the FDA, eliciting this off-the-cuff quip about the agency. "It's not easy dealing with the FDA. As soon as you say FDA, you're talking hundreds of millions of dollars. What can you get through the FDA that doesn't cost a hundred million dollars? Maybe a [PSA] test kit. At Hybritech, our

FDA problems were a fraction of those for other companies. Still it's a hundred million bucks for a test kit, I suppose."[10]

Franz Kafka very well might have placed one of his bureaucracy-bewildered characters in the FDA, trapped in an impenetrable maze of paper, red tape, and counternarratives. Its modern iteration began in 1906, when President Theodore Roosevelt signed into law the Food and Drug Act, which created the FDA. The agency tries to keep ahead of problems before they occur—from *E. coli* outbreaks to faulty hip implants—but its actions are often after-the-fact reactions that are, as was in the case of the Hybritech Tandem-R PSA assay, largely ineffectual. In fairness to the FDA, the agency is charged with regulating industries that account for about 25 percent of the nation's consumer spending, a daunting task. Nonetheless, you'll soon learn, the FDA's role in the PSA health disaster was inexcusable.

In the medical-device-approval process, products must be deemed *safe* and *effective*. However, the FDA Medical Devices Division has a checkered past, marked by a sieve-like approval process that loosed countless thousands of harmful devices into our public market. When waves of adverse events (AEs) and lawsuits began surfacing, Congress enacted the Medical Devices Amendments in 1976, establishing a three-tier approval system based on the device's potential for harm, if faulty or used off label. (An AE is any unfavorable and unintended sign—including an abnormal laboratory finding—symptom, disease, or injury associated with the use of a medical treatment, procedure, or device. Off-label use of prescription drugs, biologics, and approved medical devices means any use that is not specified in the labeling approved by the FDA.)

Class I and class II devices—from bedpans to scalpels to wheelchairs (manual wheelchairs are class I, electric are class II)—go through a comparatively easy approval process called 510(k). And once a new device is approved, a competitor can get a speedy 510(k) approval based on what's called substantial equivalence. Implantable pacemakers, brain scans, or diagnostic kits are class III, requiring a far more stringent process, known as premarket approval (PMA), in which clinical trial data are needed to support the device's claimed purpose.

On a cold, sunny morning, shortly before 9 o'clock on December 9, 1985, 14 men in business suits assembled in Room 703–727A of the Hubert Humphrey Building in Washington, DC. The group, each member of which was solicited for his expertise, were participants in the Immunology Devices Panel meeting of the Medical Advisory Committee, an FDA advisory committee; the panel consisted of four voting panel members, five consultants, three FDA representatives, and two presenters for Hybritech. After coffee and small talk they began the public hearing, the purpose of which was to discuss a PMA of the Hybritech Tandem-R PSA test kit. Following introductions, some boilerplate announcements, and an overview of the PSA kit itself, the main event got underway—clinical studies presented by Paul Lange, MD, a urologist and professor and chairman of the Department of Urology, University of Washington School of Medicine, supporting Hybritech's PMA application.[11]

A twist preceded Lange's presentation. The FDA executive secretary, Srikrishna Vadlamudi, PhD, said the purpose of the meeting was to "discuss a tumor marker kit used as an aid in the management of patients with prostate cancer." This was a mighty fall from Hybritech's original intention: developing a prostate cancer early detection test to be used on men aged 50 and older, which would be snapped up by urologists and advocacy groups as a national screening tool. But a funny thing happened on the way to the forum: Hybritech obviously did not have the supporting data for an early detection prostate cancer test, in contrast to a monitoring test. However, from a business point of view, simply monitoring men who already have prostate cancer represented a tiny and fickle market, compared with the mind-boggling prostate cancer screening market of 30 to 40 million men per year, yielding lucrative downstream procedures and drugs.

Lange, a lanky man with swept-back sandy-colored hair began his presentation with an odd, almost giddily delivered remark. "Some people say there is nothing worse than an unbeliever who becomes a believer in terms of his zealotry. So if I act a little zealous, please forgive me. I hope that I am interpreting what I have seen [the clinical nuances of data] correctly."

No matter what level of scientific understanding one has, it takes a hefty dose of denial not to be dubious about Lange's hope. The crux of his argument for approval lay in comparing PSA against another marker—prostatic acid phosphatase (PAP). Like PSA, PAP, an enzyme, is also produced in the male prostate gland. Once touted as a potential early detection tool, it is now used sparingly, if ever, as a marker in advanced cancer. So Lange, on behalf of Hybritech, faced the uphill battle of convincing a group of doctors that PSA is better than PAP. In essence, Lange was touting the worth of one marker by comparing its value to another marker whose time had since passed. That's a pretty low bar to step over, but even that small step gave Lange trouble.

Confronted with questions about his scrambled pieces of evidence, he moved on with alacrity. But he wasn't convincing and his assertions about PSA's ability to gauge disease progression were challenged numerous times during the course of the meeting. For instance, asked what might provoke a rise in PSA, Lange responded, "We are studying prostatic massage and I can tell you that with massage, PSA does go up." Even here, in 1985, at the edge of PSA's evolution, the panelists expressed unease about attaching a clinical value to a rising PSA number, given that it could be caused by factors other than the cancer itself, such as a prostatic massage.

Lange's answers to follow-up questions about PSA's accuracy in defining a change in a patient's condition did not convert the panel to his argument. If anything, the more information Lange offered, the murkier his argument about PSA's clinical value became. But the exchange that best captured the inconsistency of Lange's presentation was over PSA cut-off levels. At one point during his presentation Lange cited a PSA level of 4.0 ng/mL as a threshold. In other words, if the PSA number was 4.0 or higher, it was designated as a red flag to alert the doctor that he needed to reevaluate his patient's cancer treatment.

As Lange moved forward with his presentation, the clinical relevance of these numbers seemed to become less apparent. Panel member Alexander Baumgarten, MD, PhD, expressed concern that Lange's PSA numbers were too variable to be used as a definitive way to monitor treatment. Lange replied, "You are exactly *right*. And basically, if you want to know the truth, I mean I didn't pick 4.0, that number is . . . some kind of sacrosanct number. We could have changed the data, made it 6.0, 8.0, made it 10, anything we want. Okay?"

Baumgarten, apparently puzzled by Lange's response pressed the question. "But the purpose of [PSA], is to give us a useful marker, because if we can't do anything with it . . ." To which Lange replied, "I understand . . . if [PSA] does, in fact, predict [cancer] progression, it is useful, even though when a patient has an orchiectomy [removal of the testicles] and has recurrence [return of cancer] there is not much we can do." Despite Lange's effort, Baumgarten's conclusion was simple: "If the [PSA] number is low, we can't do anything; if it is high, there is generally no point in doing anything [because the disease has spread and the patient will likely die]."

After that exchange, perhaps out of politeness, Baumgarten left one question hanging in the air: Exactly what clinical use does this test have for a doctor treating men with prostate cancer?

Even more disturbing was Lange's response to a question by a panel consultant, Jayson Hyun, MD. "I gather you have been following patients with the PSA for several years now," Hyun said. "Do you feel that this periodic monitoring has improved the 5-year survival of your patients?" Apologizing to the panel, Lange replied, "We have not been following PSA for years. This [data] is retrospective."

The foregoing exchange is recorded on page 87 of a 106-page transcript of the Immunology Devices Panel meeting, which means—unless we are to believe that Hyun alone was confused—that for more than half the meeting, the panel members were being inadvertently misled into thinking they were viewing *prospective* not *retrospective* data. This distinction is more than medical wonkiness. Prospective trials assess patient results as they are unfolding;

retrospective trials look backward in history and are more prone to error *and* suspicion.

At the close of Lange's presentation, there were a few questions and then the panel convened in a closed-door session to hash over its approval determination for which the information was not accessible. The vote could go three ways: approval, disapproval, or approval with conditions. After an unusually long deliberation, the panel reconvened in the public room, like a jury ready to deliver a verdict. The panel chairman, Harold Markowitz, MD, PhD, said, "As you can see from the time taken, there has been quite a vigorous discussion and a number of people have been a little unhappy with the product [Hybritech Tandem-R PSA test], citing primarily the fact that prospective studies should have been done, and that the studies presented were incomplete."

Despite candidly voiced misgivings and a call for Hybritech to initiate prospective clinical trials, the four voting members decided to approve the Hybritech test, subject to *very* strict limitations. In retrospect, that decision seems counterintuitive. The evidence presented that the Hybritech PSA test helped doctors treat their prostate cancer patients simply wasn't adequate and the panel so much as said so. But sometimes, when we want to believe in something, we weave a story in our minds to shore up flimsy facts.

In 1986, the Hybritech Tandem-R PSA test was approved for use in the clinic as a tool in the management (monitoring, following) of men who had been treated for prostate cancer. However, what happened the following year began what I believe was tantamount to malpractice for profit by the American health care system. The results are still with us and it is impossible for those who participated in it to divest themselves of responsibility, including the FDA.

THREE
WHAT THE *BLEEP* JUST HAPPENED?

Well, I guess in all honesty I would have to say that I never knew nor did I ever hear of anybody that money didn't change.

—Cormac McCarthy, *No Country for Old Men*

On the way to finding the truth there is a lot of mud in the geyser between the bubbles and the smoke.

—Norman Maclean, *Young Men and Fire*

Like most stories that unspool over many years, this one has its own peculiar peaks and valleys between the milestones. This is a good time for me to pause and shift gears before moving ahead to 1987 and the event that accelerated the medical firestorm that the FDA's 1985 Immunology Devices Panel was so uneasy about. Most of those involved in the PSA story prefer to keep secret its more troubling particulars, hoping the information will just fade away among the clichéd phrases such as, "It's the best we have." For many years, that was an effective way to promote routine PSA screening in asymptomatic men (men without any obvious symptoms and otherwise healthy).

Prostate cancer's clinical vagaries are difficult for a man to grasp, especially when his mind is short-circuited by a raw fear. After hearing a diagnosis of cancer, he emerges from the doctor's office changed. Despite all our medical progress, the word cancer still boils down to an emotionally disintegrating equation: Cancer = Death. Of course, that bleak equation, made in the moment of shock, is unbalanced. Survival rates in cancer differ widely. Pancreatic cancer is usually a terribly swift journey toward death, while childhood leukemia and testicular cancer are highly curable. Prostate cancer, which kills about 30,000 American men each year, has a perplexing split-personality nature, making its diagnosis and treatment as much art as science. So before we move on to 1987, let's look at prostate cancer from the inside out, from the gland itself to the intricate aspects of the man that's wrapped around it—parts too often lost in the transition from diagnosis to treatment and beyond.

"WHY ME?"

I have few regrets in my life and most are trivial except for one that haunts me: I was unable to save my father as he was dying of prostate cancer. I continually ask myself: if I knew then what I know now, could I have found a way to stop the process that killed him? He had regular medical checkups, which, on my insistence, always included a digital rectal exam (DRE) to check for bumps or irregularities in his prostate. On one of his last visits, the urologist said his prostate felt kind of "boggy."

If you pinch the web of skin between the index finger and the thumb, you feel a spongy-like sensation, which is what a boggy prostate gland feels like. It usually indicates prostatitis and/or BPH (benign prostatic hyperplasia), the latter a bothersome age-related condition that swells the prostate. But if you touch the bone at the base of your thumb, that's what prostate cancer feels like to the gloved finger of a doctor doing a DRE.

My father also experienced increasing low back pain—a discrete symptom of advanced prostate cancer—which he passed off as sciatica from years of hard work selling and trucking premium gifts that banks gave to their new account customers. It was during an era when men complained less and trusted their banks more. I remember the first real sign that my father's body was turning against him. It was a hot afternoon in July. After playing a round of golf he stopped by my house and I noticed that his abdomen was bloated. He blamed it on a meal of bad shrimp, but when he said he couldn't urinate, I took him to Northwestern Weiss Memorial Hospital, Chicago. There, doctors catheterized him to resolve the urinary retention and told him to return the following day.

The next morning my father had a complete workup that culminated in a diagnosis of stage IV[1] (also known as stage D) prostate cancer. There was long pause as the full meaning of the diagnosis set in, and he asked me, "Why me?" As messy as life can be, it's about continuing to do things and my father's "continuing" had just been scuttled, leaving him emotionally at sea. In visual terms, his X-ray lit up like a Christmas tree—imagine the bright bulbs ringed around a tree as the cancers throughout his body. But I needed more, so I brought the biopsy slides to a pathologist friend who confirmed what I suspected: my father had the most aggressive type of prostate cancer.

My father immediately began radiation therapy, which savaged his hardy 185-pound frame. A man who could play 36 holes of golf under a blistering sun moved in tentative baby steps as though crossing a pond of thin ice. Hormone therapy, which removes or blocks the action of male sex hormones, such as testosterone, which can cause prostate cancer to grow, brought some relief; he regained a reasonably good fraction of his vitality, but then the cancer progressed and began swallowing him like a sinkhole.

In what amounted to a medical Hail Mary pass, we flew my father to the Buffalo General Hospital in upstate New York where my old colleague Maurice J. Gonder performed cryosurgery (freezing the tumor). Although conventional surgery of a primary tumor cannot eliminate advanced (metastatic) cancer, my hope was that the freezing would provoke a powerful immune response as I had seen in my earlier work. After a few days to recover we flew home and hoped for the best.

About a week later my father's pain had lessened but one day he spiked an inordinately high fever and had to be hospitalized. What I had hoped was an immune response to his cancer from cryosurgery turned out to be an infection. He remained hospitalized for about a week, during which his cancer went into a teasingly brief remission. After the hospital stay, my father began a swift decline. Even though there is no cure for late-stage prostate cancer I wanted to extend his life, if only by weeks. I gambled on a chemotherapy called cisplatinum, which has several nasty side effects, including heart damage. The cancer and the treatments had already weakened my father's heart considerably, making the decision more agonizing. Although he said, "Let me go," I was at the edge of an emotional cliff, desperate for anything that would give him more time. I prevailed over his doctor and my father was admitted into the hospital and started on intravenous cisplatinum.

There was nothing much left of him—95 pounds of loose flesh struggling to sit up. Feeling betrayed by his own body, he looked into my eyes and asked, as he previously did on learning of his initial diagnosis a little more than a year earlier, "Why me?" This is a crushing question frequently posed by people dying of cancer. As a son, I had no answer. But as a scientist I'd say, "Why *not* you?" Humans are composed of tens of trillions of cells, each one holding a spiral of DNA, a string of letters holding our life's secrets. In an oversimplification, one is a mutation that alters a normal gene into a cancer-causing oncogene resulting in an immortal cancer cell. We've identified numerous environmental and hereditary risks for cancer, but much of it, as in my father's case, just comes down to a bad roll of the genetic dice.

A few days into what would prove to be his final treatment I received a call at about 2:30 in the morning from the urologist saying that he'd just left my father and I should hurry to the hospital if I wanted to say goodbye. It was delivered with a cold sense of urgency. My father died before I arrived. He was 67 years old when his agonizing way to death ended.

YOU CAN'T HAVE IT BACK

Of the various risk factors for developing cancer, your age, pedigree, or family history rank at the top, especially in breast, colon, and prostate cancers—the closer the family member, the greater the risk, fathers or brothers being the closest ties in prostate cancer. Because my father died of prostate cancer, I am 2.2 times more likely to develop the disease than a man with no family history.

Prostate cancer essentially is a disease of aging. About 40 percent of men between the ages of 40 and 49 have prostate cancer. The rate rises exponentially to almost 70 percent in men between the ages of 60 and 69. After age 70, about 80 percent of men have prostate cancer. The common phrase, "some men die of prostate cancer, but all men die *with* prostate cancer," scratches the surface of the disease's duality.

My father died of prostate cancer. I'm 73 years old. Considering my family history and age, a Vegas bookmaker would probably lay 4 to 1 odds that I have prostate cancer. Yet I have always refused to have my PSA tested. It's not that I'm careless or apathetic about my health. I want to live as long a life as possible. But I don't want to face the PSA quandary that has forced millions of men into a clinical decision that can leave them crippled—psychologically and physically—for life. In the coming pages you'll meet an eclectic group of men who were faced with that very decision and learn firsthand how their decisions affected their lives.

The Vegas bookmaker metaphor works here because, as uncomfortable as it sounds, there is no sure thing—every decision regarding your health is based on odds, especially in prostate cancer. The personal decision not to have my PSA tested affects only me. But how can I argue unequivocally that population screening for prostate cancer is bad public health policy, a life-and-death decision that affects upward of 40 million American men and their wives, lovers, and children? In part, the answer has factors that contradict intuitive thinking. So I've honed the rationale against population PSA screening into a simple message called the *four cruxes*. I'll get to them soon.

THE PROSTATE IS A WALNUT-SIZED GLAND weighing approximately an ounce. Partly glandular, partly muscular, the prostate is located between the urinary bladder and the penis. It rests on the rectum. The urethra runs from the bladder through the center of the prostate to the penis. When men urinate, the bladder contracts, forcing urine through the prostate and out the urethra through the penis. With age, the prostate enlarges, compressing the urethra and causing different degrees of uncomfortable and embarrassing urinary retention problems. It's a democratic process, eventually affecting all men as they cross the midcentury mark, from corporate CEOs to panhandlers.

The prostate gland's chief job is to secrete an alkaline fluid (the liquid part of semen) into the urethra, contributing to the sperm's ability to move freely toward its ultimate goal: joining the female ovum (egg) and creating a human life. Anatomical illustrations, like flat-world maps, distort the interconnected reality of the body's internal landscape. The prostate's environment is clustered with networks of dense tissue, blood vessels, and the prostatic plexus, a cordlike bundle of nerves that cover the prostate, running down the penis. Called the cavernous nerves, these infinitely delicate whitish fibers made of neurons are fundamental to a man's sexual health. One can't separate sexual health from the health of the whole man. It's not just sex.

A man can live without his prostate, but once it is removed, he suffers varying degrees of physical and psychological changes. Laurence Roy Stains, author of several popular men's health books such as *Sex: A Man's Guide,* has written about this in a blunt and searing way. He captured men's post-prostatectomy angst in a magazine article called "I Want My Prostate Back."[2] Stains, in his towel-slapping locker-room vernacular, ably seizes the emotional rollercoaster of a rising PSA, which in his case had jumped to 12.9 ng/mL then went back down to 9.2. His primary care doctor sent him to a urologist. After a normal rectal exam, the urologist suspected that Stains's higher-than-normal PSA number was from an infection, which is common. He prescribed antibiotics and sent him on his way.

But the PSA number worried Stains. Once a man hears that number, worry is his main driver. Stains fixated on one thing: his PSA was higher than 4, heretofore the standard cutoff point for having a biopsy. There is no "normal" PSA number; using 4 as the cutoff point to recommend biopsy was arrived at arbitrarily.

After a few days of nerve-racking indecision, he talked himself into having a biopsy. Often dismissed by urologists as a routine procedure, a biopsy of the prostate can result in residual pain, blood in the urine and/or stool, and infection, sometimes life threatening. I'll discuss biopsy in detail in a later chapter, but for clarity, here's a brief take.

The most common type of prostate biopsy is done transrectally (passing through or performed by way of the rectum). The procedure uses transrectal ultrasound that creates a video image of the prostate to guide placement of the needle or needles. Before the advent of ultrasound, the urologist would guide the biopsy needle's trajectory with his finger in your rectum. Now, an antibiotic is given an hour before the biopsy. Then you're gowned and positioned on your side, knees bent. The nurse arranges pillows for you; she might even give you a couple of foam prostate models to squeeze as the procedure begins. Think of John Wayne biting a bullet. The urologist enters, gives the customary reassurances, gels your rectum, and does a brief finger exam. Then he inserts the ultrasound-guided biopsy gun—about the size of a roll of quarters—and injects lidocaine into the tissue surrounding the prostate (think of a dentist numbing your gums). You'll feel a sharp pinch. Then it's biopsy time.

Yes, it is a spring-action gun and it can misfire. When positioned correctly—the needle tip must be *exactly* at the target—the urologist fires, usually an 18-gauge needle, through the rectal wall into your prostate (you'll hear a mechanical *snap*). The hollow needle removes slender cores of tissue. Each "shot" is a fraction of a second. Usually 6 to 12 core samples are taken; a pathologist collects the tissue on slides for microscopic examination. Then the worst part: waiting.

After Stains had had a few days of painful urination and numbing anxiety, his biopsy results arrived: 2 of 12 cores tested positive for prostate cancer. The Gleason score was 7, putting Stains close to the cusp of the higher-risk 8 to 10 stratum. How these ten numbers add up usually signals a go or no-go decision for treatment, usually one form or another of surgery or radiation, or active surveillance.[3] This is head-spinning time for a man. First, he tries wrapping his head around PSA numbers, then a Gleason score. It's like being quantified by mysterious numbers that don't always add up in your favor.

The Gleason score, named for its developer, Donald Gleason, MD, is the gold standard used to assess the aggressiveness of your cancer. It is an old system, and it is imperfect. For one, it is largely subjective. Simply put, the system assigns cancer cells a score from 1 to 10 by combining the two most predominant patterns of cancer cells to calculate a score. In Stains' case, it was 3 + 4 = grade 7. A Gleason score of 6 or less is considered low grade; 7 is intermediate; and between 8 and 10 is high grade. Here's a simple analogy to explain what pathologists see on slides when trying to determine the grade of cancer. Imagine you're in an airplane coming in for a landing. Below you see a golf course; the fairways and greens and white-sand bunkers are neat and well organized, each with a defined border. This would represent a well-differentiated cancer. Now imagine flying over another golf course where the rough encroaches on the fairways and weeds have overtaken the bunkers and the green, an intermingled cacophony without defined areas. That would represent a poorly differentiated cancer—the degree of disorganization of the cells indicates the severity of the cancer.

Complicating the matter, Gleason scores can be affected by many external factors. Remember, this is tissue on a piece of glass that is analyzed (read) by human beings of various degrees of competency. The score is a man's critical juncture in the pathway to life-changing treatments. Most men, urged by their urologists, rush this process. But if you are confronted with this decision it is vital to take your time. Remember, you're not facing sudden death from a brain aneurism.

Still, Stains decided to have his prostate removed. The fear of the cancer accelerates and disengages the decision-making process. Think of decision making like driving a manual car. You slip into first gear, progress slowly, ease on the gas and shift into second, repeating this process until you're sailing along in fourth gear. Hearing the C-word, men fly into fourth gear and hit the gas. This C-word phenomenon is universal, even among the most well informed men. In a later chapter, you'll meet a nationally recognized oncologist and hematologist, a prostate cancer specialist, to boot, who upon being diagnosed with prostate cancer had a C-word rush to treatment, which he now regrets.

I asked the internationally regarded pathologist Jonathan Oppenheimer, MD, about the current state of prostate pathology. "The process is clearly not working to find slow-growing tumors, which we should be calling neoplasms not cancer," he said. "For instance, by calling the 3 + 3 = 6 Gleason score 'cancer' pathologists are doing a disservice to patients, by scaring them into having conditions treated that will not harm them."

He added, "Until pathologists start identifying these Gleason 6 findings as neoplasms, the harms will continue."[4] Oppenheimer explained that errors in the sample must also be taken into account. In any event, a diagnosis of prostatic neoplasm doesn't mean the patient and his doctor can let their guard down. They should continue to monitor the prostate, but there is no reason to proceed with treatment at this point.

Stains's surgeon extolled the virtues of robotic surgery, a fairly recent addition to the growing medical armory in prostate cancer. The sales pitch is easy. First, it's new, high-tech, and very expensive—a perfect fit for the American psyche. And a robot's "hands" don't tremble during surgery. Marital disharmony doesn't distract them. They don't suddenly come down with the flu. But the sexiest pitch purports that robotic surgery results in fewer of the side effects men dread most: incontinence and erectile dysfunction.

However, recently data lend little support to those claims. Robotic surgery units are very costly and need to be used frequently in order to amortize debt and start turning a profit. So centers promoting robotic surgery won't let data get in their way. Why should they? Most of what men know, or believe they know, about their health comes from the 24/7 blitzkrieg of direct-to-consumer advertising. The ads for robotic surgery often feature a middle-aged man dancing with his wife. Romance is in the air. The subliminal takeaway is: have your prostate removed by robotic surgery and soon you'll be dancing her into the bedroom.

Stains joked at one success story: his urination function returned and he was once again "pissing like a racehorse." But he wasn't the same man after the robotic removal of his prostate, and to his credit he pulled no punches talking about that: "I wonder how much of the sexual wreckage is more than just nerve damage," he wrote in *Men's Health*. "Without any ejaculate, I feel like a broken toy. Like a water pistol that squirts jelly. (Or nothing.) If love ever comes my way again, I'll sort of dread it. I'll be a spectator at my own sexual rehab, and we all know what that does for an erection."[5]

Although Stains takes care to build a comfort zone around his decision to "have it out" and offers some valuable guy-to-guy information, the meat of the message boils down to this disturbingly common internal dialogue: "Did I need surgery or not? Because if I didn't, I want my prostate back."[6] In a bid for self-reassurance, Stains asked several doctors if he'd made the right call to have his prostate removed. The uniform reply was *probably*. Seven is the "probably" number. When Stains glided by gurney into the OR and was positioned under a robot, his prostate was gone for good. And he can't get it back.

The Gleason number 7 can haunt a man for a lifetime.

THOSE PESKY FACTS

When a 50-year-old man went for his yearly physical, he routinely had a PSA test, quite often without his knowledge. The level of his

PSA could propel him into the prostate cancer industry, without understanding the potentially life-changing consequences. Notwithstanding the Orwellian ring of that phrase, the prostate gland is at the epicenter of a worldwide trillion-dollar industry and the PSA test is its kingpin. Think of PSA as oil. If the test were made irrelevant, an industry would crumble. You don't have to be a conspiracy theorist to grasp what the stakeholders will do to keep this industry booming.

Have men been saved by the PSA test? Yes, but serendipitously, which means that a certain number of men will have a potentially lethal cancer caught on the PSA road from test to biopsy. But the human toll on that overcrowded road is extremely high. Although the evidence against population PSA screening is mounting, the industry has the muscle to skillfully countermand the evidence with slick campaigns.

In 2009 the results of two much-anticipated PSA studies from the United States and Europe were published in the *New England Journal of Medicine*. Stakeholders routinely criticize clinical trials, especially hot-button studies that affect public health policy and, in the case of PSA, their wallets. But no one was able to punch holes in the studies' collective conclusion: "PSA-based screening results in small or no reduction in prostate cancer-specific mortality."[7]

In 2011, when the US Preventive Services Task Force used the two studies as the backbone of its policy recommendation against routine PSA screening,[8] it caused a furor of public outrage. The blogosphere exploded, likening the task force's recommendation against PSA screening to a slow, agonizing death sentence for millions of American men. The lay press ran front-page stories on PSA. Testimonials by men purportedly saved by PSA screening were featured on health care blogs. Prominent doctors and national prostate cancer-advocacy societies piled on with doomsday predictions of returning to the "old days when most men were first diagnosed with incurable cancer."

The president of the American Urological Association (AUA), Sushil S. Lacy, MD, said, "The AUA is outraged at the Task Force's failure to amend its recommendations on prostate cancer testing to more adequately reflect the benefits of the PSA test in the diagnosis of prostate cancer. It is inappropriate and irresponsible to issue a blanket statement against PSA testing."[9]

The task force never issued a *blanket* recommendation against PSA testing. Michael L. LeFevre, MD, cochair of the task force said, "We are charged with making recommendations about what preventive services are most likely to benefit the health of Americans and the scientific evidence we reviewed sends a different message about PSA screening than the widely held belief that PSA-driven early detection of prostate cancer is a lifesaver with insignificant harms."[10]

In a previous interview, the task force's other cochair, Virginia Moyer, MD, addressed the blanket-recommendation accusation: "The bottom line is that science tells us there is very little benefit and significant harms associated with mass routine screening. Before a man goes ahead with PSA testing, he needs to be fully aware of what he's getting into, and currently that is not how it's being done."[11]

Moyer is a reasonable and frank woman. As a primary care doctor, she's on the front lines of our health system. Her position that routine PSA screening does more harm than good has been informed by hard data, not a corporate bottom line. She leaves the door open to any man who wishes to be screened, as long as he's informed about the pros and cons and potential harms. In urology circles, following Moyer's guarded approach would turn the raging PSA river into a dripping facet.

I recently spoke with Michael Greenspan, MD, a Canadian urologist who specializes in prostate cancer-treatment-related erectile dysfunction. Greenspan, who has performed more than 1,000 penile implants, gave this frank assessment of PSA's monetary connection to American urology. "Without radical prostatectomies, more than half of all the urology practices in the United States would go belly-up."

I don't engage in psychological speculation, but it's apparent that many urologists defend PSA screening because without the test they would be pushed to the edges of irrelevance, and, as Dr. Greenspan pointed out, to bankruptcy.[12]

MORE OUTRAGE, MORE PESKY FACTS

Urologist Deepak A. Kapoor, MD, president of the Large Urology Group Practice Association (LUGPA) fumed, "We are appalled at the Task Force's recommendation that healthy men should no longer receive PSA tests as part of routine cancer screening."

Along with serving as LUGPA president, representing more than 1,800 urologists across the country, Kapoor is also chairman and CEO of Integrated Medical Professionals, a company that, among other services, helps doctors maximize their business potential. He added, "Failure to detect prostate cancer early will create a public health catastrophe in 10 to 15 years."[13]

I find it interesting that Kapoor's crystal ball predicts a looming public health catastrophe if healthy men are not routinely PSA screened for prostate cancer. What does he call millions of men crippled by unnecessary radical prostatectomies or radiation therapy? Collateral damage? I call *that* a public health catastrophe. I am not a medical fundamentalist wishing to impose my worldview on the health system, but I do wish to liberate men from the dogma and fear tactics espoused by businessmen-physicians who integrate profit into clinical decision making.

Kapoor bristled when the chief medical officer of the American Cancer Society, Otis Brawley, MD, suggested that many in the urology community promoted PSA to keep the heady revenues flowing. Kapoor countered that the notion that he would treat patients who don't need therapy was "morally repugnant." The ever-candid Brawley had more to say: "We in medicine need to look into our soul and we need to learn the truth. If your income is dependent on you not understanding something, it is very easy not to understand something."[14]

But what do the data from these trials—which have caused such uproar—mean in real-life terms? What's the takeaway message for the average man sitting in the doctor's waiting room? Here's how two impartial, nationally recognized experts interpreted the results.

Peter Bach, MD, a health care policy specialist at Memorial Sloan-Kettering Cancer Center in New York City, gave a pithy analysis of the data: "If a man has a PSA test today [2009] that leads to a biopsy and a diagnosis of prostate cancer that he is treated for, there is a 1 in 50 chance that by 2019 or later, he will have been saved from a death from a cancer that would otherwise have killed him. And there is a 49 in 50 chance that he will have been treated unnecessarily for a cancer that was *never* a threat to his life."[15]

Rightfully so, men recoil from having their personal health issues examined by some pointy-headed policy wonk as if their life were a ball spinning around a roulette wheel. But Bach—who once served as senior adviser on cancer policy for the Centers for Medicare and Medicaid Services (CMS)—made a very lucid health benefits-versus-harms equation that speaks directly to the PSA public health issue. It is about odds and how many men need to be screened and suffer the subsequent harms to potentially save one man's life.

Here, cognitive psychologist Hal Arkes, PhD, who spent his academic career exploring how decision making affects health policy, offers a more visual interpretation of the statistical results. "Most men rely on anecdotal evidence when it comes to health decisions, such as PSA screening. You know, it's the brother-in-law's experience, or promotions they read or see on TV. They don't look at the epidemiological evidence that gives a statistically precise decision. Unfortunately anecdotal evidence leads to decision-making based on emotion, not evidence."

The soft-spoken academician visually illustrated the results of the data: "Picture two auditoriums, each filled with 1,000 men. One auditorium is filled with men who had PSA screening tests, and one auditorium is filled with men who had not been tested—8 men in each auditorium will die of prostate cancer. As hard as it is for some people to recognize, these two auditoriums represent the statistical reality of prostate cancer."

To Arkes, the essentials of his comparison weren't terribly complicated. "I simply wanted to find out how the two groups of men (PSA screened or not-PSA-screened), actually fared. I found that when you compared the screened versus the non-screened groups, the men who weren't PSA-screened had a better fate than the men who had PSA testing," noted Arkes. "Among the 1,000 men who had the PSA test, 20 of them would have radical prostatectomies for cancers that never would have cause symptoms. And five of those men would have lifelong complications, including impotence and incontinence."[16]

The term *treatment* sounds innocuous, even encouraging. It implies an action that will lead to a cure or at least the lessening of troubling symptoms. You've just heard Drs. Bach and Arkes drill down into the results of two trials looking how PSA screening affects men's mortality. Now let's look at how having your prostate removed after a cancer diagnosis affects your survival.

A well-regarded study, "Radical Prostatectomy versus Observation for Localized Prostate Cancer" (PIVOT), looked at this critical dilemma by following two groups of men diagnosed with localized prostate cancer (confined to the gland itself).[17] One group had radical prostatectomy, the other group active surveillance. The researchers, a nationally regarded group of PSA-agnostic doctors, concluded: "Among men with localized prostate cancer detected during the early era of PSA testing, radical prostatectomy did not significantly reduce all-cause or prostate cancer mortality, as compared with observation [active surveillance], through at least 12 years of follow-up. Absolute differences were less than 3 percentage points [statistically insignificant]." In other words, having the surgery was no protection against dying, of prostate cancer or any other cause.

Michael Barry, MD, one of the authors of the PIVOT study told me:

> I wish we had had this information decades ago. I was involved with
> the study for more than 20 years and we found that the death rates
> from prostate cancer did not differ significantly between men who

were screened and those who were not screened. Conventional thinking is to find prostate cancers as early as possible. However, the underlying message from PIVOT was to wait and biopsy men at a higher PSA level than the current 4, perhaps higher than 10 ng/mL. Rethinking the PSA-to-biopsy paradigm could greatly minimize the unnecessary procedures and harms we currently see.[18]

THE "RABBIT" AND THE "TURTLE"

So let's now go to the *four cruxes,* which lay out much of my rationale against routine PSA screening for prostate cancer.[19]

First, PSA cannot diagnose prostate cancer. The protein I discovered in 1970 is prostate specific, *not* cancer-specific. It is present in the normal, the benign, and the cancerous prostate. And the PSA level can be elevated by a number of nonthreatening factors such as ejaculation 24 hours prior to the test, an infection, BPH, or activities that "massage the prostate," like a long bicycle ride. These potentially confusing factors are rarely part of the doctor-patient discussion. Why?

Second, there is no specific level of PSA that detects prostate cancer. This is why the current numbers used by physicians to suggest a biopsy results in a flood of unnecessary workups. In other words, a man can have a PSA level of 0.5 ng/mL and have cancer, while another man can have a PSA of 11 ng/mL and be cancer free. The biopsy cutoff level, made arbitrarily, was actually lowered at times to catch what urologists call low-hanging fruit.

Third, the PSA test cannot distinguish an indolent cancer from an aggressive cancer. Imagine a turtle and a rabbit in an open box, the box representing your prostate gland. The "turtle" is an indolent, nonlethal cancer that wanders about the box, making its hypnotically slow and endless journey to nowhere. The "rabbit" is an aggressive, unpredictable cancer—it races and hops about, it might even jump out of the box at any time. That is what happens when the cancer cells spread from the prostate capsule, metastasizing to other parts of your body.

And *fourth,* as I've mentioned, prostate cancer is age related. If a group of asymptomatic men between 60 and 69 years old have PSA-prompted biopsies, more than 65 percent will be positive for prostate cancer. So that means that a PSA-prompted biopsy may or may not, related to the man's age, find cancer. And because we are unable to determine which cancers are "turtles" and which are "rabbits," among these men, it results in a huge amount of unnecessary procedures—PSA testing essentially becomes like flipping a coin. Thomas Stamey, MD, a well-known urologist and one-time proponent of PSA, put it this way: "You can biopsy according to whether a man has blue eyes or green eyes and get pretty much the same results as biopsying according to PSA."[20]

As mentioned, the clinical problem is that we cannot differentiate between the "turtle" and the "rabbit"—that's where our research efforts need more focus. But here's the extremely salient point: despite the high rhetoric by PSA advocates, there is no evidence that proves population screening for prostate cancer extends the lives of men. And, as you've read in the previous pages, well-respected doctors and public health experts are garnering powerful evidence from clinical trials to prove that PSA screening does far more harm than good.

Remember the term *low-hanging fruit?* Well, here's the bottom branch.

Louise C. Walter, MD, a geriatrician at San Francisco Veterans Affairs Medical Center (VAMC) studied PSA screening patterns in 662,262 men at 104 VAMCs around the country. The findings were no less than shocking: On a national average, 45 percent of men over the age of 85 years with four or more serious illnesses were screened with a PSA test.[21] These are very sick men with short life expectancies who will ultimately die of causes other than prostate cancer. Yet even they are being given PSA tests. To what end?

Comprehensive cancer-center guidelines for PSA screening advise against testing men 76 years and older.[22] Medically speaking, it borders on malpractice if a PSA test given to an 85-year-old man with multiple illnesses led to a biopsy that led to a radical prostatectomy.

When I asked Walter why this was happening at the VA, she said, "No matter what the man's age or health status, he was routinely given a PSA test [in the VA system]. Although we have a better understanding of the harms associated with PSA tests in the elderly, especially those who are sick, PSA screening in the VAMCs still operates on automatic pilot, which is not a good thing."[23]

Walter's measured response begs the question: Why would doctors in the VAMCs give PSA tests to very old, very sick men fully knowing that there was no clinical benefit, just potential harm? The larger question is: where was government oversight to protect these vulnerable men—who served their nation—from this systemic and dangerous practice?

Still, the PSA proponents find a way to justify widespread screening, in what amounts to a misguided public health policy. T. Ming Chu, PhD, of Roswell Park, who held the original patent on the PSA test, made this startling remark: "If even one man's life is saved by the PSA test, the work in PSA has been a success."[24] It is that kind of evangelical belief in PSA that led us down the road to the health care disaster at the heart of this book. That said, PSA testing does have some limited value, as long as it is used properly. One way is to employ PSA as a risk-stratification tool to identify men who, because of family history, race,[25] or other identified features, are at significantly higher risk for prostate cancer than the general population.

Yet, for that approach to work the medical industry would need to reshape its biopsy-treatment, profit-driven model and recognize that the PSA test is also detecting many benign abnormalities such as prostatitis and BPH. Then, using serial PSA follow-ups from an established base line in concert with other diagnostic tests could *possibly* produce health benefits. But even tinkering with profit in the health care industry would require a cultural sea change, something that's not likely to happen any time soon.

Health care is not a zero-sum game. It is a game of educated decision making and chance—and it's best to have the odds in your favor. As noted in the four cruxes, the overriding clinical problem is distinguishing the nonthreatening "turtle" cancers from the potentially deadly "rabbit" cancers. The good news is that there are many more turtles than rabbits. But that message comes as cold comfort to men as they face a psychological tug of war after their urologist tells them, "Your PSA level is elevated, we need to do a biopsy to rule out cancer."

The question, "What do I do now?" is wedged into the mind, a constant brain ache of unease. Their doctor's advice—as their wife or partner's—weighs heavily, too. But doctors, who are trained to attack disease, face their own medical paradox: in most cases *not* treating prostate cancer may the best medical course of action. Despite the convenient lack of clarity to emerging data, doctors are beginning to come around. But as a species, they are historically slow on the uptake when it comes to some new method or way of looking at clinical issues. It's hard to break from the herd. And then insurance companies don't pay you for doing nothing, so there's that.

Bottom line: There's no *right* answer, but the last-ditch defense by the PSA-to-biopsy-to-treatment proponents that "we must do something" does not engage the issue in a constructive way. It simply uses fear to fuel the prostate cancer industry.

Statistics are cold; numbers don't reflect the flesh-and-blood sensitivities of the human experience. But the relevant point here is that we are a nation of more than 300 million people, of which 40 million are men whose age puts them at higher risk for prostate cancer. That's a lot of men and prosperous nations like ours usually abide by a moral imperative to do anything necessary to save its citizens' lives. That's a good thing; it makes us a more civil society. There's never going to be an easy way to sort this PSA dilemma out but I want you to think about this statistic—cold as numbers can be—because it does reveal flesh-and blood realities: men have a 3 percent lifetime risk of prostate cancer death, which means that 97 percent of men will have a PSA test that will probably do more harm than good. And the harms are substantial.

Advocates of PSA screening, especially prostate cancer survivors, meet what I've just said with abject scorn. They argue that if not for

PSA screening they might have been in that 3 percent, never seeing their daughter's marriage, their grandson's first birthday, or the walk on the beach they're now enjoying. These are gripping testimonials; I've heard many. But this is not about one man's story pulling at the heartstrings of policy makers. This issue is for the greater good of the American public. I would say to the advocate who makes the case for PSA screening with his personal story of survival—I'm glad you're alive, but sorry, mister, this is not just about you.

A TRAILBLAZER

You'll recall that my father's prostate cancer went into a brief remission following cryosurgery. At first I thought the cryosurgery produced an immune response that attacked his metastatic disease, bringing his cancer into a state of remission. Instead, the severe infection caused another type of immune-system phenomenon called a Coley's toxin response, after its originator, William B. Coley, MD. Immune responses, although intriguing, are fickle.

Not only was Coley a dedicated researcher, he was a doctor's doctor. Deeply moved by the death of his early patients who had succumbed to advanced bone tumors (sarcomas), Coley pored through the scientific literature looking for a clue that might lead to an effective treatment. After he found hints of a connection between infection and possible tumor regression, Coley pressed on. In 1891, he theorized that severe infection could cause an immunological response powerful enough to kill cancerous tumors. He injected streptococcal[26] organisms into one of his cancer patients, purposely creating a potent infection to stimulate an immune response. The tumor vanished, apparently from the immunological attack, which Coley had anticipated.

It was a dangerous procedure and two of his patients died of their infection, but even in these unfortunate cases the tumors had regressed. Coley saw that promise and persisted in his research. In an effort to lessen the danger he began combining the heat-treated streptococcal organism with another bacterium. This "pasteurized" version, known as Coley's toxin, was widely used for several decades. There were documented successes, but also inconsistencies in Coley's work that brought harsh criticism from his peers, especially from those in the emerging field of radiation therapy.

Still, Coley, who became known as the Father of Immunotherapy, pursued his work in the nascent field until the end of his career. From all accounts, he was a purist, putting scientific principles, no matter what the personal or professional risk, before popular opinion. We now know Coley's intuitions were correct: stimulating the immune system can be an effective way to treat cancer. Whatever was to be learned from Coley's work came to a grinding halt in the early 1960s when Congress passed the Drug Efficacy Amendment, which assigned Coley's toxins a "new drug" status, making it illegal to prescribe outside of a clinical trial.

Much of the concern about new drugs came in the wake of the thalidomide disaster, in which tens of thousands of babies, whose mothers had taken thalidomide for morning sickness, were born with horrific birth defects. With its newfound power to regulate, the FDA based its approval of new therapies on meeting a rigorous safety and effectiveness standard. Although Coley's toxins had shown promise in several clinical trials, the treatment did not meet FDA approval standards. Chemotherapy and radiation were also emerging as so-called mainstream treatments, pushing Coley's theories to the margin of medicine. In addition, Coley's toxins were dirt cheap compared to the new treatments that would soon fuel the growing pharmaceutical industry.

It would have been interesting to be a fly on the wall in the room where the FDA panel killed Coley's toxins for not meeting its safety and effectiveness standards. In a few pages you'll be a fly on the wall as the FDA makes one of the agency's most egregious mistakes. Remember the phrase "safety and effectiveness": it will reverberate in a room filled with high tensions and mute acceptance as the FDA panel rendered its decision on the approval of the PSA test.

THE GENIE'S OUT OF THE BOTTLE

I have an image in my head of men being herded into clinics or mobile vans set up to test PSA. They've taken it as an article of faith, preached by urologists, that the PSA test will ferret out cancer and lead to life-saving treatment. These men have chosen to believe their doctors, even though the doctors cannot back up their claim with scientific evidence. Throughout history, we've seen the awesome power a message has to sway large groups of people into conformity, exponentially accruing new members. Crowd psychology has been studied for centuries. It manifests in behavior as diverse as war protests to videos going viral on the Internet or, as you'll soon read, men being persuaded into having a PSA test.

I WANT TO REVISIT a couple of simple issues crucial to the next chapter. First, as I said in the four cruxes, PSA is not cancer specific. It is a protein excreted from the normal, benign, or cancerous prostate. PSA is measured in nanograms, a billionth of a gram, a unit so small it's brain-cringing to imagine. If you counted one number every second it would take you 32 years to count to a billion! As I said earlier, you can have a PSA level of 0.5 and have cancer; conversely, you can have a PSA of 11 and be cancer free. I'll discuss how we arrived at the current cutoff level in chapter 4. The cutoff has been debated over the past decades, but the current number a urologist uses after a routine PSA test to suggest a biopsy to rule out prostate cancer is 4. It's worth remembering that William J. Catalona, MD, the doctor who was largely responsible for setting 4 as the cutoff admitted that the number was arrived at "sort of arbitrarily."

As I've said, because PSA is not cancer-specific, the rise in level could be caused by a number of factors such as sexual intercourse 24 hours prior to the blood draw, an infection, a condition called BPH, or simply age. There are others, some of which have yet to be identified. So it is easy to see how unstable the PSA test is as a marker for cancer. This is not to say that PSA doesn't have clinical value; it does when used in the tightly controlled manner.

Let's go back to the stability problem.

The assay itself—a biochemical test kit that measures the presence or concentration of PSA in the blood serum—can give different readings depending upon the manufacturer and the way the kit is calibrated in each particular pathology lab. Then, of course, there's human error to factor in.

Remember the 1985 FDA Immunology Devices Advisory Panel meeting where Dr. Paul Lange pitched, with far more enthusiasm than evidence, for approval of Hybritech's PSA assay as an aid in managing men with prostate cancer? Remember how reluctant the advisory panel was to recommend approval? It was as though some members were holding their noses and casting a vote for an unworthy candidate. Given Lange's presentation it should come as no surprise that if you add an unstable tumor marker to an unstable test, it produces an unstable result. Not much for a man to hang his hat on.

Another point before I move on. The private interviews of Hybritech's executives—Howard Birndorf, Ivor Royston, and others—revealed that they always had their sights set on a strong diagnostic device that out of the gate would produce a healthy-enough revenue stream to fund Hybritech's dream, moving from diagnostic devices to the more lucrative therapeutics market. Their ultimate goal was to penetrate the big leagues of blockbuster cancer drugs.

The point being that Hybritech never visualized its PSA test to *monitor the progression of prostate cancer* in men already diagnosed with the disease. That small, difficult-to-penetrate market was inconsistent with Royston's master plan—there wasn't any money in it. Not only is the market small, but you have to convince doctors that the test helps their prostate cancer patients *and* their bank account. A tough sell on both counts.

However, the same test can capture a 40-million-men-per-year screening market. Yet Hybritech filed with FDA for a monitoring approval. Why? Obviously it didn't have the evidence for approval of a diagnostic device, which is far more stringent than for monitoring. So, according to the exchange that follows between Lange and Robert Vessella, a well-connected researcher, Hybritech gave Lange money to fund some "serious lab work"[27] of his own and sent him to the FDA with a hodgepodge of data and newfound confidence in PSA, as evident from his statement to the FDA panel: "Some people say there is nothing worse than an unbeliever who becomes a believer in terms of his zealotry. So if I act a little zealous, please forgive me. I hope that I am interpreting what I have seen [the clinical nuances of data] correctly."[28] His conversation with Vessella confirms the existence of that zealotry:

> VESSELLA: We have the serum, Hybritech has the PSA assay.
> LANGE: If [PSA testing] doesn't work (Murphy[29] and company
>   fooled us once, etc.) Hybritech was stupid to have developed it.
> VESSELLA: We need the money for "serious" [his emphasis] lab work.
> LANGE: OK.
> LANGE: [Two years later] You're right, I'm wrong, the data look
>   great.

I asked Lange to explain this exchange between him and Vessella. But Lange never responded to my e-mails asking him to clarify what, at least to me, appeared to be a scientific-gun-for-hire arrangement. He's since had an epiphany about the value of population PSA screening. Realizing that the harms outweigh the potential benefits, he has modified his recommendations accordingly and adopted a more cautious approach when it comes to suggesting a biopsy.

But speculating why doctors like Lange took so long to come around to realizing that routine PSA screening does more harm than good does not address the more important issue in this book. Millions of men have been harmed because of the misuse of the PSA test. And it continues.

Upon FDA approval, a device is issued a label indicating exactly what it can be used for. Again, the Hybritech PSA test was approved as a "safe and effective" aid in the *management of men already diagnosed with prostate cancer*. Employing the test for any other purpose would constitute what is called off-label use, posing a potential threat to patients. The FDA is charged with ensuring that all drugs and devices are being used for their approved indication. In reality, the agency is stretched far too thin to be effective and works on a sort of triage system, using its oversight power in the most effective way. Budget cuts also dilute the agency's workforce. And frankly, many of the larger pharmaceutical and device companies don't take FDA warnings too seriously; they pay the fines and continue in a business-as-usual manner.

To be clear, cancer drugs are routinely used off label, especially for patients with incurable disease. In such dire circumstances, off-label use is understandable. Even so, if physicians want reimbursement for off-label drugs they prescribe (they do since that's how they make most of their money), they must provide evidence gleaned from the medical literature validating the drug's effectiveness. No such off-label wiggle room existed for devices such as the Hybritech PSA assay. The FDA is charged with ensuring that market-hungry device companies don't violate the restrictions of their product's label, putting their own financial self-interests above public safety. We'll see how the FDA handled a flagrant disregard for the PSA test's label.

OPENING THE FLOODGATES

I previously mentioned Dr. Thomas A. Stamey. His is not a George Clooney type of fame, but he was certainly a one-time star in prostate cancer. He played a pivotal role in the early PSA story and later paid a price for his outspoken positions. He was born in 1928 in Rutherfordton, North Carolina. He attended the Johns Hopkins University School of Medicine. He left Johns Hopkins for the West Coast, where he became the chairman of the division of urology at the Stanford University School of Medicine. It was there that his long career took root. The ensuing years were punctuated with hundreds of authored papers in prestigious medical journals and awards from major medical societies. He also pioneered several eponymous surgical procedures, such as the Stamey procedure, commonly done to relieve women of stress incontinence.

Stamey, a stern-faced man in wire-rimmed glasses who favored bow ties, is forever synonymous with a paper he published in the *New England Journal of Medicine* on October 8, 1987.[30] The paper's title, "Prostate-Specific Antigen as a Serum Marker for Adenocarcinoma of the Prostate," sounds innocuous enough. Published in a dense medical journal, it largely remained invisible to the lay public until some science reporters, egged on by interested parties in the urology community, ran stories in the mainstream press. But as a scientist reading the bland, fairly ambivalent last paragraph of Stamey's conclusion, I was left in awe of the effect the article had.

Stamey's paper compared the clinical usefulness of PSA and PAP (prostatic acid phosphatase). You'll recall that PAP is the ineffective tumor marker that Lange also compared to PSA in his FDA approval presentation on behalf of Hybritech. A little more than a year after FDA gave Hybritech the green light for marketing its PSA test for managing men with prostate cancer, Stamey's paper used essentially the same weak comparison of PSA and PAP, but obviously looked for a different result.

Was the camel edging its nose under the tent, looking for PSA as a diagnostic test?

In a nutshell, this is what Stamey found after he studied serum samples from 699 men, 378 of whom had prostate cancer: "We conclude that PSA is more sensitive than PAP in the detection of prostatic cancer and will probably be more useful in monitoring responses and recurrence after therapy. However, since both PSA and PAP may be elevated in BPH, neither marker is specific." But it just took three words from the whole paper to jump off the page into the waiting arms of the urology community: "PSA is more sensitive than PAP in the *detection of prostate* cancer and will probably be more useful in monitoring responses and recurrences after therapy [emphasis added]." But the last four words of the conclusion should have tamped down the enthusiasm: "neither marker is *specific* [emphasis added]."[31]

In 1987 Stamey concluded that what I have been saying for more than 25 years is correct. PSA is not cancer-specific. But the word *detection* edged the tent flap up. Several more journal papers followed, making the case for PSA as the long-awaited early detection marker. For a while, Stamey became the poster-doctor of PSA and one of the country's lead urological surgeons, removing hundreds of prostates. The ripple effect turned into a veritable tsunami. A well-known prostate oncology specialist, Oliver Sartor, MD, from the Tulane Cancer Center, offered this explanation for the explosion of off-label PSA testing: "Everyone in cancer is always looking for ways to detect disease. Along comes the PSA test and it just ran ahead of the evidence. The mantra 'early detection saves lives' became an unquestioned truth. But nothing in medicine should be unquestioned, and PSA is a good example of that. The test just took on a life of its own."[32]

Sartor is right about PSA's surge; the national megaphone chanting the early detection mantra helped fueled it. PSA was what men were waiting for. The test's purported promise pumped up advocacy efforts. Groups like Us Too, led by charismatic prostate cancer survivors, began promoting quick, painless, and in some cases, *free* PSA testing. The public was lulled into acceptance mode; after all, aside from skin cancer, prostate cancer is the most prevalent cancer in men, second only to lung cancer in deaths. But in spite of all the promise of an early detection device that would save men's lives, the main driver of the PSA test was, in fact, money. Promoting something, even when the tactics border on profiteering, is hard to challenge when the stated end goal is saving men's lives.

Peter Albertsen, MD, who has an international reputation for his work in prostate cancer, shed light on the post-Stamey explosion of PSA testing. He noted that urologists saw the test as a huge moneymaking opportunity, which became a centerpiece of the urology business model. "Even though the test has limitations, sometimes people don't want to look too hard at a gift horse,"[33] said Albertsen. The physical ease of the new test helped the promotion. "Overnight, a procedure that did not require booking into a hospital basically became a no-brainer. It became a test that takes 15 minutes, with no pain, and is relatively risk free," he noted.[34]

The psychology of marketing medicine is based on the principle that there's nothing as immediate or personal as health. Even in bad economic times, it's an irresistibly tempting market. People of all ages and social strata obsess about finding the next medical development that will help them live longer and better lives. But there's an even stronger motivator: making money. When asked if he still had the drive for more money after making his first million at Hybritech, Birndorf scoffed at the concept of enough: "What's enough? I mean, I don't know. I'm still driven by making money; I'm still driven by having toys and nice things. It's not as much anymore, though. It's different. How many cars can you have? How many houses can you have? It's not the same anymore. I really do things now because I really like them . . . it's still a thrill to put something together and to get it to work, and get the money, and the people, and the deals, and everything."[35]

Urologist Joseph Oesterling, a doctor at the epicenter of the PSA explosion, said the main driver of widespread off-label PSA testing was the inundation of grip-and-grin industry sales reps persuading doctors to integrate PSA into their practices. "They went around the country saying 'Doctor, you need to get a PSA on your patients. Start using it. Start using it.' The next thing, patients started coming in and saying, 'Doctor, check my PSA.'"[36]

In 1989, as the wind behind PSA testing gathered force, an advocacy group called the Prostate Conditions Educational Council launched its first Prostate Cancer Awareness Week. The council promoted free or low-cost screening sites across the country, the first of many such programs. On the surface, it all seemed good. Advocacy groups raised lots of money and awareness. They became highly polished lobbyists, glad-handing and arm-twisting their way through the power corridors of Capitol Hill, for a cause nobody would dare challenge. In fact, the Best Practice Committee of the National Alliance of State Prostate Cancer Coalitions published a manifesto in 2004 that includes the edict "Recruiting is Selling. It's a SELLING job."[37] It may be tempting to connect industry, advocacy groups, and pols in some backroom arrangement to lube the gears of "the big prostate cancer machine." It happened, but not like that. There was no grand collusion—just a lot of self-interested groups vying for all the money and power they could leverage from the nation's $3 trillion health care system.

For instance, since the breakout of PSA testing in the late 1980s, advocacy groups have become a big business in their own right. Set up like corporations, they need heavy revenues to pay themselves and to pay for their activities, such as celebrity golf tournaments that raise cash to fund PSA-screening drives. After a while, the front people running large advocacy organizations begin to look a lot like the powerful and wealthy entities that support them.

An advocacy organization called ZERO: The End of Prostate Cancer, headed by the magnetic CEO Skip Lockwood, a prostate cancer survivor himself, has 55 corporate sponsors. It's a who's who of pharmaceutical heavyweights, among them Beckman Coulter and Abbott, market leaders in PSA-test kits. Another group is international organization called Us Too, which unabashedly displays its 25 corporate supporters in cash-cow categories designated by precious stones and metals. The leading supporter is pharmaceutical powerhouse Sanofi Oncology, sole occupier of the Diamond category. Next is Platinum, where Dendreon shares a berth with Novartis Oncology. There are categories for Emerald, Sapphire, Gold, down to the lowly Friend category. Most Us Too financial supporters have lots of skin in the prostate cancer game.

When Hybritech's Tandem-R PSA assay was approved for monitoring men with prostate cancer it opened the floodgates for the off-label PSA screening I've described. Undeterred by any potential FDA crackdown on off-label use, other companies (Abbott for one) jumped onto the PSA-test bandwagon, grabbing huge chunks of the market from Hybritech. This didn't sit well with Hybritech's parent company, Eli Lilly, which would soon be trolling the waters for potential buyers. In all fairness to Hybritech, Abbott's sales force is considered second to none in the aggression department, noted for its willingness to do almost anything necessary to get the sale.

Abbott is an example of how, left unchecked, the medical and pharmaceutical industry puts profit over patients. In 1997 Abbott formed a joint venture with a Japanese drug company, TAP Pharmaceuticals. TAP had the drug Lupron, which the FDA approved for use in treating prostate cancer. Lupron suppresses testosterone, the hormone that fuels the growth of prostate cancer cells. Despite the terrible side effects that men endure—enlarged breasts, hot flashes, weight gain, loss of libido, and urinary problems—TAP's sales force put a full-court press on the urology market. Although the FDA indicated its use for prostate cancer, urologists began prescribing Lupron to men simply because their PSA was elevated. Doctors could not get enough of it, especially since Lupron was so well reimbursed by Medicare. Then some whistleblowers exposed TAP for dishing out generous cash kickbacks to urologists for prescribing Lupron. On top of that, TAP was charged with illegally inflating Lupron's wholesale price, bilking Medicare and American taxpayers out of millions of dollars. It's a dirty story, ending with TAP paying out the largest-ever civil and criminal settlement in health care fraud history: $875 million.[38] It's worth noting another odd twist to the TAP scandal; although the company paid a huge settlement for defrauding the government, TAP employees were later acquitted at trial. The TAP venture dissolved, but Abbott went on, celebrating its 125th anniversary this year. There's a surreal amount of money at stake—Big Pharma companies simply pay the fine, no matter what the transgression, and move on.

By 1992 PSA screening was peaking, becoming an accepted screening tool for more than 30 million men a year. The test was a dream come true for the medical industry, especially the urology community. But what about the effect its use had on men? In 2009 Gilbert Welch, MD, and Peter Albertsen, MD, analyzed data from the National Cancer Institute (NCI) to assess PSA use from 1986 to 2005. They found a rapid increase in prostate cancer incidence, which makes sense, since the more men you screen the more cancers you detect. But as we know, most prostate cancers are harmless. According to Welch, since 1986 more than a million additional men were over-diagnosed and unnecessarily treated for prostate cancer, a conservative estimate made even more alarming when you consider that he stopped analyzing PSA data almost ten years ago.

"But the number that really sticks out is in younger men. . . . We found more than a seven-fold increase in prostate cancer incidence in men younger than 50. It's worth noting that during part of the period we looked at, the cut-off number was reduced from 4 to 2.5 ng/mL. Every once in a while I think you need to include the unit of measure for the reader. The lower the cut-off, the more biopsies you get," Welch told me during an interview, adding, "We also estimated that for each man who had a presumed benefit, more than 20 men had to be diagnosed with prostate cancer."[39]

In 1994 Eli Lilly finally found a buyer for its beleaguered Hybritech division. Lilly never really understood the diagnostics-devices business and was glad to unload its ailing subsidiary to the device maker giant Beckman Coulter. The financial deal between Lilly and Beckman Coulter doesn't add to the story. But what juiced up the deal for Beckman Coulter does. Although sales for the Hybritech PSA test were limping along, Eli Lilly was about to apply for a new indication as an early detection device for the diagnosis of prostate cancer. If approved by FDA, the Hybritech PSA test would be the first and only test in the world *approved* as a screening tool. It was a long shot. And to have a chance, it needed to bring in someone who had a stake in the prostate cancer industry, a doctor I have publicly debated on the misuse of PSA.

THE RADICAL

If you happen to need an operation, medical data indicate that quantity matters—so make sure your surgeon has a lot of experience before you go under the knife. Few surgeons, if any, have more experience in prostate cancer than William J. Catalona, MD, who by his own count has performed more than 6,000 radical prostatectomies—the PSA test is the conduit to his scalpel.

Catalona has long been the go-to surgeon for well-heeled men with prostate cancer; he deftly uses his celebrity patients such as baseball greats Joe Torre, Stan Musial, and Bob Watson to bullhorn his PSA message. In 1992 then US Senator Bob Dole called Catalona out of the blue and thanked him for his efforts to get out the PSA message, which Dole credited with saving his life. Dole even gave Catalona a red-carpet tour of the Capitol, introducing him to well-connected members of Congress who pledged support for increasing PSA awareness. A remark by Republican Senator Jeff Sessions captured the zeal-over-reality zeitgeist of PSA promoting congressmen. "They draw blood, may check your cholesterol and PSA at the same time. If that comes back positive, they can do a biopsy that will confirm the PSA," Sessions said.[40] Dole's own prostate cancer story is best remembered for a series of cringe-worthy self-effacing Viagra commercials that stirred more than 750,000 letters from thankful men, many of whom said that Dole's story had convinced them to get PSA tested.[41]

Despite the growing amount of evidence showing the overwhelming harms associated with routine PSA screening in healthy men, Catalona remains an unyielding promoter of the test. Short and slightly built with hair that over the years has turned as white as his lab coat, Catalona soldiers on through photo ops with professional athletes and TV spots with a smile. Still, the data are clear: PSA screening leads to unnecessary life-altering procedures. But for Catalona to acknowledge that many of those 6,000-plus men may have had needless surgery would be overwhelming and humbling. After all, he has preached the benefits of PSA testing and the radical prostatectomy for more than four decades—he has announced no plans to modify his approach.

Since the mid-1980s physicians around the country held to a rule: do not biopsy men with a PSA level less than 4 ng/mL. In 1995 Catalona led a study in which 332 men who had PSA levels of between 2.6 and 4 were biopsied, finding that 22 percent of the men had prostate cancer. Of course, we don't know whether the cancers were "turtles" (nonaggressive) or "rabbits" (fast growing). Regardless, citing his own study, Catalona began biopsying all his patients with a PSA of 2.5 or higher, noting that the study results emphasize the need for yearly PSA tests. "All it takes is a simple blood test. It's so easy, and it *may* prolong lives [emphasis added]," said Catalona.[42]

He put his decision to lower the biopsy number into perspective during an interview in the *New York Times*. Catalona, who was then director of the Prostate Cancer Program at Northwestern University, took credit for being the primary mover behind the widespread interest in PSA screening. When pressed, he agreed that the test wasn't cancer specific, but "we were willing to pay the price."[43] What about the price paid by the men who were left impotent and in diapers? Of the journal papers dealing with various PSA issues I've reviewed over the past 30 years, few, if any—for example, a recent study by Johansson et al[44] being one—have taken a penetrating look at the long-term psychological effects (that is, silent versus mechanical) of impotence and incontinence or what those words mean to a man in the bedroom or walking down a fairway with his buddies.

In the early 1980s, when Catalona was making his argument for PSA screening at the NCI, he remarked that he was "howled down" because the NCI was looking for something as specific as a pregnancy test. "When it's positive you always had cancer and when it was negative you never did," he said. In hindsight, the NCI seemed on the right side of this issue, but it lacked the gumption or authority to call attention to a disaster in the making.

An exchange with a *New York Times* reporter underscores the reality of Catalona's private prostate cancer world. Asked how the PSA cutoff number of 4 for biopsy was determined, he conceded that it was adopted "sort of arbitrarily."[45] This perplexing response begs me to ask: If the number 4 was arrived at arbitrarily, was lowering the cutoff to 2.5 also arbitrary? Why not 1.5 or 0.5 . . . why not just do a biopsy on *every* man of a certain age?

Catalona discovered early on that simple messaging could serve as the raw material for his PSA promotional tour. His scientific slide presentations often ended with take-away warnings such as "If you are a healthy man aged 40 to 69 who does not want to die of prostate cancer, *there is conclusive evidence that PSA testing can save your life* [his emphasis]." He ended that presentation with a cartoon of an old man at the Pearly Gates saying to St. Peter, "I'd have been here sooner, if it hadn't been for early detection."[46]

Catalona's stature in the urology community and his continued PSA-screening promo tour paid off in the form of a mutually beneficial relationship with Beckman Coulter/Hybritech, which lasts to this day. The company funds Catalona's research and pays him consultant and speaker fees for promoting their diagnostic devices, most notably, of course, their PSA test(s). Catalona and Hybritech's marriage (while fully disclosed) is a stark example of the business-as-usual conflicts of interest that have plagued our health care system. I'll return to this important discussion later, but for clarity, as I'm using the term, a conflict of interest in medicine is any situation in which an individual with responsibilities to another (financial or otherwise) might, out of self-interest, consciously or unconsciously prefer one outcome to another. Furthermore, a conflict can exist even if it is fully disclosed.

And when something—even something as insidious as flouting the trust between medicine and patients—is so commonly pursued, over time it tends to become opaque to the public eye. Most important, it exists largely because the FDA, America's safety watchdog, denies or refuses to put the uncomfortable facts about these self-serving and destructive insider deals before the American public. It's a form of complicity by default.

THE MEETING

It was an unseasonably warm Tuesday morning on June 29, 1993. The Plaza I Ballroom of the Holiday Inn Crowne Plaza in Rockville, Maryland, was quiet save for the chinking of coffee cups being stacked and the workaday chatter of busboys. The open public hearing of the Immunology Devices Panel[47]—an FDA medical advisory committee—would hear evidence to approve or disapprove Hybritech's PSA test for the early detection of prostate cancer. A decision that would affect more than 30 million men annually.

Peter Maxim, PhD, the executive secretary from the FDA, asked the 15 panel members (only nine were voting members) to introduce themselves and then read the FDA's conflict-of-interest statement, which "addresses conflict of interest issues associated with this meeting and is made part of the record to preclude any appearance of a conflict." Besides a few grants and speaking honoraria, none of the panel members reported any conflicts worth noting.

I found Maxim's closing comments solicitous and, given the circumstances that first encouraged me to write this book, insulting. He said, "But what we have to do is post-market surveillance or post-approval studies that will allow us [the FDA] to observe if the approved device, when released into the general population, has a diminution in its effectiveness."

Translation: the FDA has an obligation to ensure that approved devices are safe and effective in the open market.

It was an empty promise, pure lip service. Where was the post-market surveillance after the FDA approved the Hybritech PSA test in 1986? Put aside for a moment the long-running debate over PSA's value; the FDA allowed device makers and the urology community to run wild with off-label use.

Maxim then turned the meeting over to chairperson Charles T. Ladoulis, MD, who opened the floor to the public hearing. The prostate cancer advocates and their supporters stirred like leaves hit by a gust of wind. After yawning through the pro forma presentations the public was finally going to get its say. Advocacy groups play a role in boosting cancer awareness; however, I've never seen their value in a scientific meeting whose purpose is evaluating a drug or device. They inject a burst of emotion into a process that should be driven by data and fact. But make no mistake, when cancer survivors talk about their struggles, the universal empathy and fear of cancer grabs people everywhere, across all social strata.

The first advocate, Jim Wise from the Robert J. Mathews Foundation for Prostate Cancer Research, said with religious conviction that PSA screening was vital for men *age 40* and older. "Since we don't know what causes prostate cancer, the only chance we have is early detection . . . reports downplaying the need for PSA screening are certain to ensure that almost a half a million men could easily die." Putting his emotions on stage reminded me of astronomer Carl Sagan's remark when he refused to speculate about life elsewhere in the universe. When the interviewer pushed him for an answer based on his gut feeling, Sagan relied, "But I try not to think with my gut."

To his credit, panel member Alexander Baumgarten, MD, PhD, asked Wise a penetrating question: "You stated that the only chance for cure of prostate cancer is early detection. If we can . . . assume that there is no specific treatment, would you still advocate detection [PSA screening], bearing in mind that, if I may use a frivolous analogy, it is rather like advertising a sale in a store that is empty?"

Wise gave a rambling nonanswer. Baumgarten repeated his question, with more emphasis. Wise acknowledged the "thrust of the question," adding, "that's very difficult, especially for us who see the realities of this disease." Panel member Harold Markowitz, MD, seized on Wise's self-regarding remark, commenting, "You've been speaking from the point of view of the victims of prostate cancer. At the same time, you don't know how many men using PSA will have false-positive tests, and will be subjected to a biopsy, which is painful and costly. What about this group?" Wise deflected Markowitz's concern saying that he'd be glad to provide the panel with dozens of letters from "victims who were detected with prostate cancer solely by a PSA test."

This brief encounter is telling on a couple of levels. First, even before the scientific presentation, it indicates the panel's unease about "relabeling" Hybritech's PSA test. Queried on the suffering of countless numbers of men harmed by PSA false positives, Wise circled the wagons around his insular community—men who claim they were saved by PSA screening—in essence, seemingly implying that their lives outweigh the harms to other men produced by false-positive PSA results. This is the common emotion-based type of exchange used by advocates to promote PSA screening. It's the kind of flag-waving patriotism that people are loath to challenge; we've seen the results of that sheeplike mentality.

There were other testimonials from cancer survivors, most notably from the advocacy organization Us Too. I only wish that I'd been allowed to present at this meeting on behalf of the million-plus men left maimed by unnecessary procedures. Those men deserve an advocate, too.

Then Ladoulis introduced the next speaker, Steven H. Woolf, MD, PhD, science adviser for the US Preventive Services Task Force. In an interview, Woolf portrayed the atmosphere over PSA screening as "highly polarizing," describing himself as "a youngster, a few years out of my medical training." He confided that he felt his age didn't lend the gravitas needed to be persuasive on such a controversial issue. Age aside, Woolf's testimony, to my mind, made an undeniable case against routine PSA testing. He opened by clarifying that the hallmark of the task force methodology is developing recommendations based on objective scientific evidence in determining which preventive services should be recommended. "Such an approach has become necessary because too many groups had promoted screening policies that lacked evidence of benefit, but carried known risks to patients and costs to society," said Woolf, adding, "Many groups that encouraged screening had a political or financial interest in promoting the recommendations and ignoring the potential harms and costs."

With this, Woolf captured what I've been saying for three decades. Remember, he's a doctor with a background in family medicine, deeply concerned about public health. He works for a nonpartisan governmental agency, with no ax to grind, and, most importantly, no financial ties to any entity that could influence his position. Woolf stated unequivocally that financial and political interests motivate population screening, thus, putting profit over the welfare of men. It's important to note that the task force relies on a sophisticated analytic methodology to determine the societal impact of population screening.

Woolf explained that the task force does not consider a screening test effective unless there is evidence that it accurately detects a condition earlier than without screening, and that the early detection improves patient outcomes. *Moreover, the benefits of screening must outweigh the potential harms associated with false positives.* This sentence spotlights the moral dilemma posed by routine screening and the impasse created by PSA proponents. How many men must suffer unnecessary harm to save one life?

Ironically, Woolf addressed this moral question by using the very data that Hybritech's "consultant" Dr. William J. Catalona was about to present. "If one uses the rates [percentage of false readings] reported by Dr. Catalona . . . the positive predicative value of PSA screening is only 1.9 percent. That means that at least 50 men with elevated PSA will undergo unnecessary workups for every man with clinically significant cancer," said Woolf. In short, 50 men run the risk of being left impotent and wearing diapers to *potentially* save one man.

Harvard biologist Marc Hauser explored this moral quagmire in *Moral Minds: How Nature Designed Our Universal Sense of Right and Wrong.*[48] Hauser's dilemmas looked at numbers, too. A typical scenario might involve a subject—call her Mary—at a switch-point on railroad tracks. A train full of people steams ahead toward a stretch of tracks that's been washed out by a storm. Unless Mary throws the switch and diverts the train to a safe track, dozens aboard will die. Here's the moral problem. An unconscious man is lying on the track that the train will be diverted to. Should Mary throw the switch to save dozens and doom one? PSA advocates use the same moral rationale in reverse. They make the case that even though many PSA-screened men will have unnecessary treatments and subsequent harmful side effects, they're alive, but the one man might die of prostate cancer if he had not been screened.

It's a fallacious argument on many levels. But Woolf wasn't finished. "It *might* be worth subjecting this many men [50] to unnecessary treatments if we knew that one man with cancer would benefit from early detection. But this leads to the second problem with PSA screening: lack of proven benefit. There is simply no evidence that early detection of prostate cancer improves the health of patients. Studies are underway to answer this question."

I've reviewed the results of the studies Woolf alluded to and, as frustrating as it is, those studies confirm today what he articulated two decades ago—there is no evidence that PSA screening or early detection improves men's health. Equally important, men treated for their prostate cancer on average do not live any longer than men who forgo treatment. And, emerging research indicates that a growing number of men, when given the unvarnished facts about treatment side effects, are opting out of having surgery. Addie Wootten, a clinical psychologist at the Royal Melbourne Hospital, framed a problem that urologists want kept in the closet: a sense of losing one's manhood. "Even men who are not sexually active in their 70s and 80s talk about how it changes something. There is an identity or core feeling of being a man that changes."[49]

Woolf summed up his powerful presentation by noting that recent studies (those about to be presented to the panel) suffered from serious design flaws, confirming once again that there was no evidence that screening improved health outcomes in men. He reiterated the single message that scrapes the nerve endings of advocates who use the deaths of thousands of American men from prostate cancer as a fulcrum for championing PSA:

> There is a tendency to want to do something to prevent this disease even if there is no proven benefit and even if it means ignoring potential harms. There is also a tendency to dismiss the physical and psychological harms that screening imposes on millions of healthy men and the billions of dollars in potential costs for the sake of those with actual disease. Although this is an understandable viewpoint for advocates of screening, it is not a sound basis for making public policy.

In the Q&A that followed Woolf's presentation, Glen P. Freiberg, an industry representative for the FDA, asked, "I have just a very brief question, because of overwhelming curiosity. Just yes or no will do. I was curious if you had ever received a report back with your own PSA value?"

Woolf replied, "No."

Woolf was finished. That was 20 years ago.

A VESTED INTEREST

Jules Harris, MD, is a longtime colleague and acquaintance of mine. He's had a fine career as a medical oncologist, serving as a board member for many prestigious associations. He's currently winding down from the rigors of his long medical road, now serving as a clinical professor of medicine at the University of Arizona College of Medicine in Tucson. I'm a professor of pathology at the U of A, so we see each other occasionally. Harris is soft-spoken, a nice man to talk with. I don't make a habit of talking shop while socializing, but I made an exception for Harris. He's long known about my passionate and vocal opposition to the misuse of PSA and my never-ending combat with the power brokers in the urology community. When I first told him about my intention to write this book, he was very supportive.

After a few conversations, Harris's own passion about the PSA scandal surfaced. Not one given to hyperbole, he said that exposing the truth about PSA's misuse and the subsequent profiteering by the prostate cancer industry was the biggest medical story of the past 30 years. But it was FDA's failure to act in the best interest of the American public that was particularly troubling. Harris should know all about that: he was one of the voting panel members at the meeting you've been reading about.[50]

The next presenter at the FDA meeting was a representative from the AUA, James E. Montie, MD, a prominent urologist who was awarded the AUA's Distinguished Contribution Award in 2007. He wasted no time stating that the AUA strongly supported PSA screening for early detection of prostate cancer in men aged 50 and older. After ticking off the usual prostate cancer facts and figures, Montie noted that black men have a prostate cancer death rate two to three times higher than their white counterparts. To which he added,

"Therapeutic nihilism, evidenced by implying that early detection is not needed, commits us to a tolerance of this acceptable degree of suffering." Translation: If you question the value of routine PSA screening, you're unsympathetic to men, especially black men, who are suffering and dying of prostate cancer.

Montie continued making his case for PSA but not without contradicting himself. For instance, he said unequivocally, "PSA is the most effective single method of detection of prostate cancer." Then, moments later he acknowledged, "Explicit data affirming benefit [of PSA screening] for prostate cancer are really not available now, as mentioned earlier [by Woolf] and these data will not be available for another 10 to 15 years." He closed his presentation by warning the audience that even though "good and bad" cancers will be detected, leading to some unnecessary treatments, the solution is "appropriate selection of the groups most likely to benefit from early detection." He also revisited the race card in, to me, language that was condescending, lecturing the audience about the need to provide free PSA screening to the unfortunates in our society. "PSA will need to be made available to individuals that may not be able to pay for it. Without this [government program], it will further disadvantage the African-American man who is least likely to be able to afford to pay for the test himself."

Montie's triangulation on routine PSA screening was contested in a spirited exchange during the Q&A. My U of A colleague Harris challenged Montie to clarify his call for routine screening, an idea that Harris, rightly so, found dangerous. Harris asked, "Are you saying that PSA testing should be used in healthy men over the age of 50 . . . who have no symptoms?"

Montie answered, "We are stating that the PSA test is useful for the early detection of prostate cancer."

Harris responded, "But you are not answering my question. Are you saying that the AUA supports the use of PSA in all men 50 and older who are healthy and have no symptoms?"

After several rounds of similar back and forth, Harris tried to corner Montie, "Dr. Montie, I want to pin you down on this. Are you saying that asymptomatic men 50 years of age and older ought to be screened uniformly?"

Montie still managed an awkward political dance around the question, but Harris had opened the can of worms. Following Montie, NCI representative Peter E. Maxim, PhD, read a statement, the operative phrase being, "There is currently no data showing that early detection of prostate cancer by PSA . . . reduces mortality or morbidity from this disease."

It's hard to exaggerate the magnitude of the potential public health care crisis Harris and others on the FDA advisory panel were concerned about. Only someone living in an alternative health care universe would not be aware that the PSA test had been misused as a screening tool shortly following the first approval in 1986. So the next presenter, FDA's scientific adviser, Raynor N. Appell, PhD, must have been met with understandable doubt when he said, "Since its approval in 1986, the PSA assay has come into wide usage and is now the standard-of-care in monitoring patients after radical therapy," completely skirting the issue of rampant off-label use. Naturally, mentioning that greed-driven companies were purposely flouting the PSA test's approved use would finger the FDA's total failure at post-market surveillance. Unfortunately, Appell's comment went unchallenged.

It is of interest that Appell took time to point out that the three formats of the Hybritech PSA assay could have slightly different readings. For example, he said, "A comparison of the three (Tandem-R, Tandem-ERA, Tandem-E) shows that the Tandem-R test gives a value slightly lower than the other two, so a sample near the cutoff of 4.0 nanograms per millimeter could read negative with the Tandem-R and positive with the other two." Appell proceeded across this rocky terrain with a "pass the potatoes, please," nonchalance that, for lack of a better term, is disturbing. After all, he had just acknowledged that the Hybritech assays are unpredictable; the reading of one model can be higher or lower than the other. Add this factoid to other the things that can confound the PSA reading—recent sex, strenuous physical activity, infection, a lab technician screw-up, etc.—and it's plenty easy to engender healthy scientific skepticism about the accuracy of the Hybritech PSA test.

It is baffling how the variance issue in test results rendered from different test kit models was given short shrift in the panel presentation. More problematic was the panel's passive reaction. A few years down the road, William J. Catalona addressed this problem, pointing out that early detection relied on two standard ways the tests are calibrated: the World Health Organization (WHO) and Hybritech. In short, Catalona noted that studies indicated that the WHO tests yield approximately 23 percent lower PSA numbers than Hybritech tests. Using a 20-million-man screening population, Catalona asserted that—because of the two tests' variability—more than 10 million men per year were receiving widely different results. "Prostate cancers could be found 1 to 2 years later in men who got their results from the WHO-calibrated test rather than the Hybritech test."[51]

So, the results of your PSA test depend on which of two ways the kit is calibrated. Without explaining why the discrepancy exists, Catalona insisted that the Hybritech test, which is calibrated to give a higher PSA number leading to many more biopsies, is the one you should insist on. At the bottom of the page, in small print, Catalona cited his financial ties with Beckman Coulter, the company that produces the Hybritech PSA test.

LET'S TAKE A BRIEF SIDE TRIP and look at this disquieting mechanical hiccup in human terms. Men are putting their lives on the line based on a test result that varies from model to model, measuring units in billionths of a milliliter. So, depending on how the test model is calibrated—lab technicians can also screw this process up—a man's PSA might erroneously be 4.1, putting him in the so-called gray zone (a PSA level of 4 to 10). His urologist might very well say, "Let's do a biopsy, just to be safe."

There are more than 1 million ultrasound-guided transrectal needle biopsies performed on American men each year. I don't know of data that would give us a "safer than driving a car" type of comparison, but, as I discussed earlier, all invasive procedures carry risk. Medical risks are calculated by multiplying the odds of something happening times the costs of the experience, both in human and monetary terms. But lines on a graph don't tell the story of the medical experience. And, reports from around the world are cataloging an alarming trend: increasing numbers of men are becoming seriously ill from potentially deadly antibiotic-resistant bacteria contracted during transrectal needle biopsy.[52]

Shane Greenstein, PhD, a 50-year-old professor of economics at Northwestern University, had a needle biopsy that nearly cost him his life.[53] Ten hours after the procedure, Greenstein went to the local hospital's emergency room in Evanston, Illinois. ER doctors gave him IV fluids to stabilize his blood pressure and prevent shock. It took three courses of antibiotics, the last by IV, to save Greenstein from the sepsis that was killing him. Since the biopsy needle "drags" bacteria from the bowel into the prostate and back out again, it can contaminate the bloodstream, as it did in Greenstein's case. Although it is common practice to administer antibiotics prior to the procedure, there is a global rise in infections that cannot be successfully treated with current drugs, posing a significant threat of deadly biopsy-driven infections.

I'm a scientist, not an alarmist. Even though the majority of needle biopsies are unnecessary, it is still a relatively safe procedure. That said, men need information in order to weigh the very real risks involved in a needle biopsy. The FDA website publishes medical device adverse events (AEs) on a dedicated site called MAUDE (Manufacturer and User Facility Device Experience). There are literally hundreds of pages of reports. Here are two examples reported verbatim from the MAUDE site:

Event date: 01/27/2009

Event Type: Injury

Event Description:

During the prostate biopsy procedure, the physician had to guide the device using a finger in the patient's rectum. An initial biopsy was taken with the physician's finger still in place. When the physician attempted a second biopsy, the needle passed through the prostate and through the physician's finger. The physician retracted the needle and removed the device. The procedure was aborted.

Event date: 01/24/2010
Event Type: Injury-Hospitalization
Event Description:
It was reported that within two days after a biopsy was performed, the patient presented with signs and symptoms of an infection. These symptoms included fever, chills, shakes and pain on urination. The patient was admitted to the hospital and received intravenous antibiotics. According to the user facility, all standard sterilization procedures were employed. The source of the infection remains unknown.

I TAKE THIS DETOUR on biopsy infection to illustrate that at the critical FDA meeting the medical language should have been scrutinized since it pertained to the health and well-being of millions of men.

After Appell finished his unchallenged explanation of the variability of the three PSA test models, he spoke about two other issues that the agency wanted the panel to pay special attention to in their deliberations. The first was the *intended* use of the test, and it was here that Appell waded into a quagmire of semantics, bringing the two terms *early detection* and *screening* into the debate. The second was the issue of false positives, which will play a dramatic role at the end of this section. Briefly, Hybritech's studies that were reported by their paid consultant, Catalona, had an inordinate amount of false positives. Simply put, the test was wrong a lot more than it was right.

Appell closed his presentation.

The chair opened the Q&A and before he finished his sentence, Harris immediately jumped in, asking for clarity on the early detection-versus-screening language. Misuse of language in medicine, especially in public health, can have grave consequences, as Harris pointed out to FDA functionary Appell. Harris said, "I think it is unwise and imprudent to use the term 'screening' for the use of

PSA . . . because of the connotation that as a test it would lead to early diagnosis and improved survival. I know of no evidence that suggests that it [PSA testing] impacts survival."

Appell tried to brush this off as simply a definition-of-terms issue. Harris was unrelenting, emphasizing the danger of using the term *screening*. Think of population screening this way: There is a peculiar malady that affects a very small percentage of girls in the age range of 3 years to 17 years. There is a newly developed medication that taken routinely *might* prevent the malady from occurring, but this medical roll of the dice comes with real side effects, some of which could be severe. Should every girl in that age range in the country take the medication? Would you want your daughter to?

Before we move to Hybritech's presentation and the dramatic conclusion of this historic meeting, I want you to hear Harris's prescient warning, spoken directly to Appell and the FDA. After what amounted to a bunch of grandstanding from various participants, Harris got in the last word. "What I want to avoid is this panel giving out the impression to the American public that this is a test which should now be used in all 30 million to 40 million men in the United States that are 50 years and older on an annual basis . . . it will overwhelm us in terms of financial costs."

COMPANY MEN

Before we move to Hybritech's presentation, I can't let Harris's best efforts pass without a recap. Woolf and the NCI's data couldn't be challenged: there was no evidence to support the use of routine PSA screening in healthy men. All the data presented thus far suggested that the promotion of routine PSA screening was based on self-interest and hubris and that it carried a danger for us all.

Next up was Hybritech's vice president of clinical and regulatory affairs, Ms. Van Johnson, who restated the history of the company's PSA test and the proposed indication as an aid in the early detection of prostate cancer. Then Hybritech's manager of clinical affairs, Katie Smith, MD, reviewed the performance data of Hybritech's three

PSA test formats stating that two of the three have been on the market since 1986 and 1987, respectively. She then stated that under the relabeling of this FDA review, there were no plans to change any of the "components or the procedure." Smith went on to say: "In conclusion, we presented data which represent the performance characteristics which we feel are important for early detection." Her conclusion about Hybritech's PSA tests' value in early detection seemed bolstered by what she called the "seven-year proven product performance in the hands of many, many customers." Proven performance of what measure? Again, the only approved indication for the PSA test was in 1986 for *managing* men with prostate cancer, so unless she was referring to the well-documented off-label use, I'm not sure how Hybritech could make this claim. More than anything, her comments provide a window into the inner workings of the next presenter, Catalona.

He opened with a boilerplate conflict-of-interest statement, listing the several layers of financial support Hybritech provided him, as a speaker and consultant. He singled out the speaker fee he received for presenting PSA research at Hybritech in 1991, which was the underpinning of his presentation at the meeting. Given the enormous consequences involved in this meeting, let's pause before Catalona's presentation and revisit the issue of industry's influence over the FDA approval process.

The former editor in chief of the *New England Journal of Medicine,* Marcia Angell, MD, addressed the conflict-of-interest problem in *The Truth About the Drug Companies: How They Deceive Us and What to Do about It* and in an editorial for the *Journal of the American Medical Association,*[54] in which she wrote, "The pharmaceutical industry has gained unprecedented control over the evaluation of its own products . . . companies now finance most clinical research on prescription drugs, and there is mounting evidence that they skew the research they sponsor to make their drugs look better and safer." Angell went on to say, "Sponsoring companies have become intimately involved in all aspects of research on their products . . . often designing the studies and performing the analysis."

And, in the case of Hybritech and Catalona, the company had an intimate relationship with the doctor who ran the trial, wrote the subsequent paper, and made a presentation to the FDA.

Catalona's presentation began with an overview of prostate cancer. He made his statements boldly, citing data from slide after slide. Panel members I spoke with described him as "very much in control of the room." Woolf, who presented on behalf of the government task force, told me that he was overshadowed by Catalona's don't-mess-with-me presence. During his presentation Catalona even took the *New York Times* to task for questioning PSA. "Here is another article from *The New York Times* . . . the message that they were trying to give us was look at the alarming increased incidence of prostate cancer detection because we're doing PSA testing, but it's not having any effect on mortality. So you're detecting more cancers but you're not curing more."

Catalona dismissed the article's spot-on grasp of the issue. Then he said, "I called the reporter from *The New York Times* and I said, 'You are a bright young woman and it is a very prestigious job being a reporter for *The New York Times*, but the down side of what you're saying is that there is going to be a man out there walking around with a lethal cancer who is going to read your article and decide not to get a PSA test today. That, I think, is an awesome responsibility." Translation: By reporting scientific evidence, the journalist just consigned a man to death.

Before we move to the second part of Catalona's presentation—the trial data that is the meat of Hybritech's case for approval—I want to point out two issues from the first part of his presentation. He revisited the pregnancy analogy, noting, "If a woman has a positive pregnancy test, you know she is pregnant, 100 percent . . . if the test is negative, you know she is not pregnant. Not so with the PSA test." Given that there is no 100 percent certainty of any test, Catalona seemed to be setting the panel members up for a type of word-and-data salad that can be tossed into a viable reason for approval, even though the test, by his own admission, doesn't do what it purports to do. Catalona asserted, "If a man is 50 years old or greater but his PSA is between 4 and 10, you immediately know that his risk of having prostate cancer is 25 percent to 35 percent on initial or follow-up biopsy."

(Remember, prostate cancer is age related: autopsy studies show that men between the ages of 50 and 59 have a 45 percent chance of having prostate cancer. Men between the ages of 60 and 69 have a 65 percent chance, *regardless* of their PSA score, of having prostate cancer.)

Catalona then stated, "PSA is not a diagnostic test for prostate cancer. It is a risk assessment test. One does not have to proceed to biopsy, even."

True, one does not need to proceed to biopsy, but biopsies and treatments are the cash cows for urology practices. The central economic elements of supply and demand are in play. For example, there are more are than a million prostate biopsies performed each year on Medicare beneficiaries, most of whom are 65 years of age or older. Because of their age, these men already have a 65 percent chance of having prostate cancer with a very low chance of it becoming aggressive. Seventy-year-old Medicare beneficiaries have an 83 percent chance of having prostate cancer. And the PSA test opens the door for that vast and highly vulnerable group of men.

Then there's the FDA label. According to the agency, Hybritech was seeking permission to add the indication "as an aid in the early detection of prostate cancer." Catalona took pains to explain that the PSA test is a risk-assessment instrument, not a diagnostic or early-detection tool. However, there is no mention on the FDA label about PSA being a risk-assessment tool. Speaking about risk, a recent study in the *Journal of Urology* found a significantly increased risk of serious infections in Medicare beneficiaries following prostate biopsy.[55]

Catalona began the second part of his testimony by saying, "I will now present the results of the prospective clinical study of the Hybritech Tandem-R PSA test for the early detection of prostate cancer." There is no benefit to the story for me to microanalyze the specifics of the trial Catalona presented, but to maintain the continuity of related events, let's hear the purpose and makeup of the study from its author. Moreover, he made some interesting observations that are worth mentioning. "The main objective of this study was to compare the effectiveness of digital rectal examination and PSA for early prostate cancer detection. In every other trial of PSA test that has ever been done, you had to have a PSA elevation and one other abnormality before a biopsy was triggered . . . it was considered unconscionable to biopsy a man just because he had an elevated PSA."

Unconscionable is a very powerful word. In legal terms, the word *unconscionable* refers to something harsh and shocking to the conscience; that which is so grossly unfair that a court will proscribe it. The doctor-patient relationship is, in fact, a contract. In contract law, an unconscionable contract is one that is unjust or extremely one-sided in favor of the person who has the superior bargaining power. This contract is one that no person who is mentally competent or, in the case of PSA, fully informed, would enter into and one that no fair and honest person would accept.

By Catalona's own admission, PSA is not cancer specific and is not a diagnostic measure. Further, again by his admission, the cutoff number of 4 ng/mL used to indicate an abnormal PSA reading was arrived at "sort of arbitrarily." Despite these facts, the unconscionable clinical behavior of suggesting a biopsy solely on basis of an artificial number has become a standard screening practice. Midway through his presentation, Catalona stated that since the introduction of PSA testing, the proportion of men with advanced, incurable prostate cancer is "dramatically going down" because of earlier detection, a central argument advanced by Catalona and other proponents of routine PSA screening.

Harris interrupted Catalona, "But you have no clear cut evidence of that [PSA's role]. It could just be greater awareness and more additional rectal examinations on patients over the age of 50."

Catalona played both ends against the middle, responding, "Right, absolutely . . . but PSA is playing a big role, both directly and indirectly." Interestingly, he never addressed Harris's concern that the facts he was laying out about PSA's role in early detection were not backed by data. But Harris wasn't satisfied. Telling an FDA panel that PSA testing reduces the number of men with incurable prostate cancer is a huge claim; he wanted evidence, not hearsay. "You're talking anecdotal impressions . . . I'm not sure the case is being made that the PSA is impacting upon this stage migration," said Harris, expecting a data-driven answer about, among other issues, his concern over stage migration. Simply put, when you screen large amounts of younger, otherwise healthy men, you detect prostate cancers, most of which are harmless. When those men migrate into the set of unhealthy men with aggressive prostate cancers, it statistically increases both lifespans, creating a misleading impression that men who undergo PSA screening live longer.

Instead, Catalona doubled down on the anecdotal evidence, throwing his surgical street creds into the mix. "I do 200 to 250 radical prostatectomies a year and my patients come from all over the country. When they come, I get their complete clinical history, and I would say that in two-thirds of my patients, their cancer was detected by PSA. I talk to my colleagues and they are sort of seeing the same thing," said Catalona, essentially closing the door on further inquiry. But before moving on, Harris had one more "to be continued" parting shot. "I have a lot of respect for that, but I have a lot of respect for data as well."

Catalona made some declarative statements in his closing remarks. I want to address them before moving to the meeting's dramatic conclusion. In confidence, one panel member told me that as the meeting drew to a close, it felt like Catalona was lecturing them, bordering on condescension. For instance, Catalona said, "One thing that strikes me is that most of the opponents of PSA screening are people who don't treat large numbers of prostate cancer patients. Although I have respect for their research, having worked with prostate cancer patients for 20 years, I've seen the agony . . . and it always bothers me to have somebody get up and say that this [PSA screening] is not a worthwhile endeavor when they have never seen a patient die of prostate cancer." He added that patients must be given the options (informed consent) so they can make their own quality-of-life decisions instead of biostatisticians making life-and-death decisions.

I'll let Catalona's words speak for him, but I'll also add a remark or two. In essence, Catalona averred that unless you've been at the bedside of a man dying of prostate cancer, you somehow lack the authority to make a scientific analytical decision about PSA's value as a screening tool. To me, that's analogous to a fireman telling a group of forensic fire investigators that it bothers him having people who haven't raced into a burning building make a determination about how the fire started or how to prevent similar fires in the future.

Then take a look at one of Catalona's more nuanced observations about the need to make educated decisions about PSA screening without being unduly influenced by biostatisticians. "I think that patients must be given the options [clinical risk versus benefits] and they can make their own quality-of-life adjustments," said Catalona. The problem with that observation is that men got swept into the "early detection leads to a cure" psychic tsunami and the only information they were receiving about PSA screening was from the urology community and advocacy groups.

Catalona also exhibited his bunker mentality at the meeting, castigating those who question routine PSA screening as dilettantes who have never "seen a man die of prostate cancer." In fact, one distinguished panel member, Sheila Taube, PhD, told me that Catalona approached her during a break—obviously upset by the panel's tough questions—and snapped, "You've never seen a man die of metastatic prostate cancer!" In fact, her father had recently died of metastatic lung cancer, a long and painful death. "I was outraged that Dr. Catalona should think that he somehow had a monopoly on the suffering created by cancer," said Taube.

From the start, Catalona and other heavily invested proponents of screening have demonized those who question screening. But it was the explosion of mass screenings in a healthy population of men that began to cause alarm in other sectors of medicine, doctors who were on the front lines of health care. From the onset of PSA screening, prostate cancer detection increased at a rate never before seen in

American medical statistics. The reported incidence rose a shocking 25 percent from 1990 to 1991.[56] The medical community was beginning to question the consequences of this kind of mass screening on uninformed men. But the voices of reason that tried to slow the process down were drowned out by those chanting the "screening saves lives" mantra. Flash forward to 2012 and have a look at an excerpt from an article titled "Uniformed Consent: Mass Screening for Prostate Cancer" in the journal *Bioethics*:

> No one would deny that a man undergoing surgery for prostate cancer has a right to informed consent. So too, however, does a man being screened for that disease have a right to be informed of the *known liabilities of the screening test itself—in particular, that it may or may not decrease mortality, often detects cancer of questionable significance, and may lead to unnecessary surgery.* Yet "in screening . . . informed choice is not common practice." In the United States, where prostate cancer "awareness" has been vigorously promoted, it is thought that a majority of men over age 50 have been screened for the disease . . . 20 years into the PSA revolution, and its generational consequences have not been discussed in the medical literature.[57]

Catalona concluded his presentation with another revealing comment. "PSA is a more powerful predictor of prostate cancer than rectal examination. A biopsy should be considered if either the PSA is elevated or the rectal exam is suspicious," said Catalona, apparently contradicting his previous statements about PSA being a risk assessment tool in conjunction with digital rectal exam—as per the FDA approval Hybritech was seeking. And, Catalona summed up his presentation with this dark warning. "The medical dictum 'at all costs, do no harm' has a corollary, and that is, if you know how to do good and you don't do it, it's a sin."

Catalona then advised the panel to approve the PSA test, saying, "This test works. The public knows it, the doctors know it. . . . I would urge you to approve it."

BEFORE VOTING, there was an open committee discussion. Not surprisingly, Harris led with the first question, prefacing it with a remark that seemed to praise style over content. "Dr. Catalona, you gave a superb presentation and you marshaled the data in a very magisterial way. It was a pleasure to listen to you and I think we all learned a great deal. You are a very effective spokesman for the urology community and for the industry you represent." It's worth noting, that Harris commended Catalona as an effective spokesman for urologists and the industry he represented, but patients were not mentioned. Then Harris asked, "But are you recommending that every male at the age of 50 years and over in the United States have an annual DRE and PSA?"

Without hesitation, Catalona replied, "I really am. I think that if they are concerned about having prostate cancer . . . the best chance of giving them an accurate answer is to do a PSA test and a rectal exam."

Harris, obviously concerned where this was going, followed quickly, "You're not recommending it [PSA] just by itself, though, of course."

Catalona countered, "Well, to tell you the truth, I think it may come to that, but I don't want to open that can of worms."

The can of worms had already been opened by FDA's original approval in 1986. What Harris and his fellow panel members were worried about was the lid being ripped off the can of worms and given a big stamp of approval on its label by the FDA.

The discussion shifted as Catalona fielded some softball questions, which gave him another opening to highlight the special needs of high-risk groups, particularly the African American community. He advised the panel to recommend that men with a family history of prostate cancer and African American men should begin annual routine PSA screening at age 40. Several minutes later, when the discussion moved into the important distinction between early detection and screening, Catalona gave these revealing observations.

When you say that PSA should be used for early detection, basically you're saying that PSA can help detect prostate cancer at an early stage. Is that going to translate into a mortality benefit? [Will men live longer because of PSA?] We don't know . . . but when you say PSA should be used for screening . . . the screening test has to pick it [prostate cancer] up early, and the early pickup has to translate into a mortality benefit . . . well, we don't have any data to show that PSA translates into a mortality benefit.

Make a note here: Catalona has just stated unequivocally that there was no evidence that the PSA test that he was advocating for had any mortality benefit. In other words, there are no data indicating that using this test extends men's lives.

Panel member Alexander Baumgarten, MD, PhD, then read from an American Cancer Society addendum questioning the efficacy of the PSA test, before asking, "The question is whether the benefit is to be confined, as I believe you've maintained, to the mere fact of detection or to the whole process of what do I do with this detection and what comes after?"

Baumgarten simply asked Catalona to explain how, considering the absence of data, PSA extends the lives of men who undergo the test and subsequent procedures.

Catalona answered, "Well, that is an excellent question and I don't know how to answer it. I know in my heart what the answer is to it. I think that we're going to cure more prostate cancer patients, but if pressed to provide data on that, I can't begin to."

Baumgarten was clearly rankled by Catalona's "from the heart" answer, which prompted this exchange:

BAUMGARTEN: "If PSA is going to be recommended to this vastly
    increased number of people . . . whether or not that procedure
    has really meaningful consequences. Otherwise you are going
    to have a heck of a lot of people subjected to a very marked
    procedure with a big question mark after it . . . is PSA a benefit?
    Or is this a national disaster?"
CATALONA: "Those are legitimate questions and I don't really mean
    to downplay them. We've been here for 8 hours—100 men have
    died of prostate cancer while we've been here."

BAUMGARTEN: "I'm sorry, sir, but this is really pejorative. You really are putting an emotional thing into what is an important question."

CATALONA: "No, I'm not. I'm saying that the issue you raised is of major magnitude, and I acknowledge that and I don't disagree in any way. On the other side of the issue, if we put our heads in the sand and don't use it and adopt a nihilistic approach [there's that word again], there are going to be a half a million men who die of prostate cancer before the PLCO study is done."[58]

BAUMGARTEN: "But the argument is that these people would have died regardless. You are making this assertion on the basis that we have something to offer."

CATALONA: "That is your opinion."

BAUMGARTEN: "No, I'm sorry. You are saying that we do not have any proof either way, and then you are saying that they [men] are going to die because we do not decide your way. That does not follow. If we do not know, that's the end of the matter. They may die regardless of what we do. You have conviction, but not proof."

Baumgarten's searing line of inquiry was abruptly cut off by panel chair Ladoulis, who somehow felt that Baumgarten was straying from the purpose of the meeting. Industry representative Glen Freiberg seconded his concern.

Let's distill what we've just heard from Catalona. He presented the data from a trial funded by Hybritech that he conducted on behalf of Hybritech. Thus far, according to questions and statements by several members of the FDA's advisory panel, the data were not only unconvincing, but in fact left more questions unanswered than answered. By Catalona's own admission, there was no evidence that PSA screening in healthy men improved their survival.

Catalona also agreed that there were significant harms associated with PSA population screening, but he contended that despite the lack of evidence and the harms to men, PSA must be approved for early detection of prostate cancer. Why? Because in his heart he knew it was the right thing to do. Remarkably, the foundation of Catalona's argument on this awesome decision faced by the FDA was based on his own private emotion. Baumgarten, fearing a national disaster, challenged Catalona's repeated emotional retorts when asked to back up his claims with data. "You have conviction, but not proof," said Baumgarten, cautionary words that went unheeded.

WHEN THE MEETING RECONVENED, Ladoulis announced that after the panel members made their final comments, the voting would follow. The panel members had three options: vote to approve with recommendations, vote to approve without recommendations, or vote not to approve the application. The first comments were reappraisals of Catalona's presentation, which, given Baumgarten's heated exchange, tended to be little more than perfunctory nit-picking, ways to be relevant without bringing the PSA pot back to boil.

Baumgarten read excerpts from several published studies, augmenting his previously articulated concern. One study he read concluded, "PSA mass screening resulted in a huge increase in the number of radical prostatectomies. There is little evidence for improved survival outcome in the recent years' comparison of data between 1983 and 1987 versus 1988 to 1992, showing a possible decrease in the five-year cancer survival rate in age groups less than 60, 60 to 70 and over 70." Baumgarten summed up his comment period with this ominous admonition: "We cannot, like Pontius Pilate, wash our hands of guilt. We must accept the consequences for what we are doing and that is creating a large number of people subjected to radical prostatectomy who will be adversely affected in large numbers."

Harris seconded much of Baumgarten's observations and added a caveat to the proposed FDA label. He wanted any statement about annual PSA screening in men 50 years and older to be omitted entirely, stating, "Because that would just be leaving the entire health care system open to a screening procedure for all 34 million American men 50 years of age and older . . . I don't think that on the basis of the information we have that it is justifiable."

I'll end the comment period with remarks by panel member Harold Markowitz, MD, PhD, who was the chair of the 1985 FDA meeting when Hybritech sought its first approval. I'm not a psychiatrist, so I don't do psychological autopsies on people, but Markowitz's remarks are filled with latent urgency.

> I'm afraid of this. If it is approved, it comes out with the imprimatur of the Committee . . . as pointed out, you can't wash your hands of guilt. I was bothered by a lot of things, like the false-positive rate of 78 percent. I have never seen this in any submission to the FDA . . . all this does is basically threaten a whole number of men with a prostate biopsy . . . it's dangerous. It's costly. But basically what has been said is, if we get one patient with cancer let's not worry about the couple hundred others who have to undergo the cost, the suffering . . . that's about all I have to say.

Ladoulis then asked, "For those who would recommend approval of this submission without conditions, please raise your hands."

There was no response.

Ladoulis then asked, "For those who would recommend approval of this submission with conditions?"

The nine voting panel members raised their hands.

Ladoulis concluded, "Then it is unanimous that the recommendation of this Advisory Committee to approve this submission with conditions," and adjourned the meeting.

On August 25, 1994, the FDA notified Hybritech that its PSA test was approved as an aid in the early detection in men aged 50 years or older. The panel's recommendations about imposing strict conditions were ignored. There was no mention of risk assessment or the panel's warning about the harms associated in screening 34 million healthy men 50 years or older. In the United States, the "screening saves lives" mantra was still drowning out the opposition in the PSA debate. However, reaction from Britain—where screening criteria are much stricter than the United States—was highly critical. For example, Malcolm Law, an epidemiologist at the Wolfson Institute of Preventive Medicine at St. Bartholomew's Hospital Medical College, said, "The decision to approve the use of PSA as a screening test in healthy men is extraordinary. PSA may detect early cancer in healthy men, though there is virtually no published evidence, but evidence from a randomized trial that such screening saves lives is essential. PSA should only be approved as an effective screening test after there is evidence available to show that it is, indeed, an effective screening test and that such screening can save lives."[59]

THE TESTIMONY YOU'VE JUST READ speaks for itself. Markowitz's declaration that he was afraid "of this" because, for one, the incredible 78 percent false-positive rate of the PSA test would condemn huge numbers of men to unnecessary life-changing therapies, is, in itself, a compelling enough argument against approval. Markowitz was a highly regarded physician who had been a long-standing FDA advisory board member, yet he was verily astonished, saying, "I have never seen this in any submission to the FDA." Yet, despite no evidence of benefit and much evidence of potential harms to men, the panel voted to approve the Hybritech PSA test. After reading the previous several pages, I imagine you'll find that panel's decision as inexplicable as I do.

Susan Alpert, MD, PhD, was the director of the FDA's Office of Device Evaluation in 1994, when the PSA test was approved for early detection. After leaving the FDA, Alpert went on to a lucrative career as a consultant for companies like the international device giant Medtronic. On January 23, 2013, I e-mailed her a simple question, one that not only deserves an answer, but one that *must* be answered.

The FDA's criterion for approval rests largely on establishing that the device is "safe and effective." I asked Alpert how could a device with a shocking false-positive rate of almost 80 percent be judged effective? Then I asked, given the well-known harms associated with such high false positives, such as unnecessary surgery, how could the device be judged safe?

Keeping those questions in mind, when the FDA made its fateful decision to approve the PSA test as a screening tool, the Agency knew—from my early observations and from studies done by the very researchers associated with the development of the test—that PSA does not detect prostate cancer.[60]

So, I will also pose those questions to the current FDA Commissioner Margaret Hamburg, MD. The answers, Dr. Hamburg, should not be lost in the obscure hierarchies of the very government agency charged with safeguarding the American people from predictable medical harms.

FOUR

THE COLOR OF MONEY

Facts do not cease to exist because they are ignored.

—Aldous Huxley

That which can be asserted without evidence can also be dismissed without evidence. . . . Perhaps you notice how the denial is so often the preface to the justification.

—Christopher Hitchens

Have no respect whatsoever for authority; forget who said it and instead look at what he starts with, where he ends up, and ask yourself, "is it reasonable?"

—Richard Feynman

The Cold War was so named because the two major powers, the United States and the Soviet Union, had enough nuclear weapons between them to assure mutual annihilation. For the most part it was a bloodless war of high rhetoric and saber rattling. The circumstances that brought the Cold War to a close are complex. But the free-spending nuclear arms race was a central factor, and that part was won handily by the United States. In short, the United States' robust free-market economy gave President Ronald Reagan much deeper pockets than his communist counterpart, President Mikhail Gorbachev.

Speaking at a Politburo meeting before traveling to the historic meeting with Reagan in Reykjavik, Iceland, Gorbachev said, "We will be pulled into an arms race that is beyond our capabilities. . . . If the new round of an arms race begins, the pressure on our economy will be unbelievable."[1]

In accord with many health care experts the United States is engaged in a medical arms race—much like the arms race of the Cold War—wasting huge chunks of our health care budget on technologies and drugs that create profit for industry without equivalent medical benefit for consumers. About 30 to 45 percent of the growth of health care spending is driven by the adoption of new medical technologies produced by the drug and device industry.[2] As evidenced by the excerpts from the FDA approval hearing quoted in chapter 3, the Hybritech PSA test was approved despite a lack of evidence. The Congressional Budget Office has reported that, "though estimates vary, some specialists believe that less than half of all medical care is based on or supported by adequate evidence about its effectiveness."[3] Moreover, in 2011, when Donald Berwick stepped down from his post as Medicare administrator, he gave this final salvo, saying that 20 to 30 percent of health care spending—more than $1 trillion a year—was waste.[4]

The medical industry spends an incredible amount of money creating these technologies and even more advertising them, using clever psychological marketing ploys to influence consumer habits. For example, pharmaceutical powerhouse Pfizer produced a sales document revealing the naked truth about Big Pharma's rapport with doctors and investigators who publish scientific papers. The omniscient Pfizer voice asked: "What is the purpose of publications?" The answer: the "purpose of data is to support, directly or indirectly, the marketing of our product." Or in short: "Purpose of publications: The bottom line."[5]

Like the former Soviet Union, the US health system is reaching a critical tipping point. Our medical spending is approaching $3 trillion per year, almost 18 percent of our nation's total gross domestic product (GDP). Virtually every health care expert, on both sides of the aisle, agrees that bourgeoning costs are engulfing our precious national resources—it's an anaconda swallowing a small deer whole. And while no single entity is the source of the problem, each must accept its share of blame. As we'll see in this chapter, public enemy number one is the self-perpetuating profit-before-patient ethos. Anthony Zietman, MD, a nationally regarded radiation oncologist, neatly framed the issue in an interview. "Today, many medical technologies are developed looking for a clinical question to answer. It's the classic case of a hammer looking for a nail. In radiation we went from having one therapy to at least a half dozen."[6]

One might reasonably ask, isn't cutting-edge innovation that brings new medical technology to the market a good thing for health care consumers? The answer is yes, but only if new technologies entering the market have proven benefit over the ones they replace.

For sheer cost and size, the flagship of the medical arms race is the proton-beam-therapy center, a huge, incredibly expensive investment for our health care system. But are the centers worth their extraordinary price tag?

Let's take a look.

RADIATION CONJURES MIXED EMOTIONS; it's an invisible force that kills and cures. The iconic mushroom clouds over Hiroshima and Nagasaki are imbedded forever in the human psyche. There were the Cold War depictions in novels and movies of radiation as a world-ending power sweeping in clouds from continent to continent. And yet, radiation is an essential part of our health care, detecting cavities, broken bones, and tumors.

The field of radiation therapy began to grow in the early 1900s, largely due to the work of the Nobel Prize-winning scientist Marie Curie, who discovered the radioactive element radium in 1898. After a storied life, from laboratories to the front lines of World War I, Marie Curie died on July 4, 1934, from aplastic anemia, believed to have developed from her long-term exposure to radiation.

Simply put, radiation therapy kills malignant tumors by damaging the DNA in the cancer cells using two types of energy—either photons or charged particles, such as protons. Like other therapies I'll discuss, proton therapy advocates use men's fear of incontinence and impotence as a marketing ploy, contending that these dreaded side effects are far milder with the enormously expensive proton therapy than with surgery or other forms of radiation treatment.

Precision is the operative term in proton marketing. Proton centers advertise that protons can be controlled and targeted, delivering the greatest amount of radiation directly into the tumor. This, they say, allows patients to receive higher doses of cancer-killing energy with less damage to the surrounding healthy tissue than standard X-ray radiation therapy. ProCure, a network of proton-beam centers across the nation claims that the extra dose from standard X-ray radiation that inadvertently radiates healthy tissue is equivalent to several hundred thousand dental X-rays. ProCure referenced several published studies to support their interesting analogy, but I'm not sure where the "several hundred thousand dental X-rays" came from. That said, the visual image of lying in a dentist's chair wearing a lead apron, with a bitewing cutting into your gums as you wait for the ominous little bzzz, does work. It sounds bad.

Unlike X-ray radiation treatment, proton-beam therapy is a form of electromagnetic energy. It is made up of particles (protons) that are accelerated to near the speed of light in a machine called a cyclotron. During treatment, the beam of protons is energized to specific velocities, which determines how deeply in the body the protons will deposit their maximum energy. All tissues are made up of molecules, atoms being the building blocks. At the center of each atom is a nucleus; negatively charged electrons orbit each nucleus. Energized protons passing through the tissue attract the negatively charged electrons, pulling them out of orbit. This process is called ionization; it changes the characteristics of the molecules within the cell, especially the DNA, or the cell's genetic material.

Damaging the DNA destroys the cell's ability to divide or proliferate, and if the damage is too extensive, the cell can't repair itself. Although both normal and cancerous cells go through this process, cancer cells have less ability to repair molecular injury, and thus sustain more permanent damage and die more frequently than normal cells. The radiation oncologist can accelerate the protons to specific velocities and determine precisely how deep to deposit the maximum energy into the designated cancer volume. Theoretically, this process causes significantly less injury in the healthy cells surrounding the tumor.

There are currently 11 proton centers operating in the United States with 12 centers in development. These football-field-sized facilities cost upward of $200 million to construct. The gantry alone—the device for rotating the proton-beam delivery system around the patient during treatment—is a three-story-high structure. According to a study in the *Journal of the American College of Radiology,* "Given the cost and debt incurred to build a modern proton facility, impetus exists to minimize treatment of patients with complex setups because of their slower throughput. Financing a modern proton center thus requires treating a case load emphasizing simple patients [prostate cancer] even before operating costs and any profit are achieved."[7] In other words, without a steady influx of prostate cancer patients, these sticker-shock-priced treatment centers will go belly up.

And despite the hype, there is no evidence that proton therapy is any more effective than less expensive radiation therapies. According to health policy expert Ezekiel Emanuel, MD, an adviser to the Obama administration,

> The higher price would be worth it if proton therapy cured more people or significantly reduced side effects. But there is no evidence showing that this is true, except for a handful of rare pediatric cancers, like brain and spinal cord cancer. . . . It is impossible to keep all . . . the proton beam centers in full use, much less the approximately 20 others in planning . . . with so few patients . . . to generate sufficient revenue, proton beam facilities need to treat patients with other types of cancer . . . the biggest target so far has been prostate cancer, diagnosed in nearly a quarter of a million men each year.[8]

He adds, "[T]here is no convincing evidence that proton beam therapy is as good—much less better than—cheaper types of radiation therapy."[9]

Since the world's first hospital-based proton-beam center was built in 1990 at the Loma Linda Medical Center in Loma Linda, California, authorities have noted that there is no proven clinical advantage over other, far less expensive therapies. Medicare pays more than $32,000 per prostate cancer patient for proton-beam therapy compared with about $18,000 for standard X-ray therapy.

As far as side effects, although proton therapy advocates tout less incontinence and impotence, again, there are no data to support the claim. A recent study published in the *Journal of the National Cancer Institute* shored up the growing data refuting the proton industry's incessant and threadbare claim. The authors analyzed two groups of Medicare beneficiaries, each consisting of more than 27,000 men. One group had proton-beam therapy, the other had a less expensive radiation treatment called IMRT (intensity-modulated radiotherapy). The researchers concluded that although proton-beam therapy was considerably more expensive, the clinical benefits were the same and the side effects were no less bothersome than the much less expensive IMRT.[10] If you parse through all the data-speak that buzzes between policy wonks and health care experts, the bottom line is there is no evidence that proton-beam therapy is better or less toxic than other, far cheaper radiation treatments.

Private insurance companies aside, why would Medicare pay for an exorbitantly priced treatment that has no proven benefit over a far less expensive treatment? The quick answer is that our nation's health care system has no cost-effectiveness strategy built into spending or reimbursement. For instance, if the FDA approves a cancer drug, no matter what the cost is relative to its effectiveness, Medicare and private insurers are essentially obligated to pay for it. Consequently, we pay more per unit of health care than any other industrialized nation in the world, often without getting our money's worth. I'll go into more detail a bit downstream.

But let's get back to the proton-beam centers sprouting up across the country. Despite the promise of an exotic new cure—it shoots a sniper's beam of invisible particles into a prostate tumor—proton therapy is a vastly expensive hype job when it comes to prostate cancer. But without prostate cancer, what's to become of the dozens of $200 million proton beam centers? Zietman thinks that centers are racing to build proton-beam centers while the Medicare reimbursement bank is still flush, then "recoup their investments by cashing in on the lucrative prostate cancer market."

Zietman asserted that it is nearly impossible for a proton facility to amortize its debt unless most of the cases it treats are prostate cancer. I asked Zietman a simple question: According to current research, what happens if Medicare reimbursement for proton-beam therapy is reduced to the level of other equally effective treatments? "They all fail," he said, adding, "This is a high-stakes game, and it boils down to prostate cancer and Medicare reimbursement."

It also boils down to this: $200 million proton-beam centers are being built around the country despite no clinical evidence that proton therapy is more effective than other far less expensive radiation treatments. Moreover, there is no clinical evidence that treating prostate cancer with proton-beam therapy extends men's lives. As Zietman pointed out, without the routine PSA screening of 30 to 40 million healthy men, the steady influx of prostate cancer patients dries up. The cash cow dies and so does the multibillion-dollar proton-beam industry.

I, ROBOT

The Renaissance titan, Leonardo da Vinci, is considered one of humankind's greatest and most diverse geniuses. Renowned in his own time as a painter, sculptor, architect, musician, mathematician, engineer, inventor, anatomist, geologist, cartographer, botanist and writer, Leonardo left an indelible footprint on our planet. I wonder how he might feel about having his name and legacy used by a company called Intuitive Surgical to brand a high-tech piece of equipment. Their da Vinci Surgical System uses prostate glands as a chief part of its revenue stream.

Since Intuitive Surgical went public 13 years ago at $9 a share, it has been embraced as the latest Wall Street darling, another Silicon Valley superstar promising a new technology that would revolutionize surgery. In its IPO filing, Intuitive crowed that da Vinci's technology was so advanced that it "overcomes many of the shortcomings of traditional surgery,"[11] with less blood loss and faster recovery.

In little more than a decade, Intuitive Surgical has exploded, its stock climbing from $9 to more than $500 per share. This past fiscal year the company's revenue topped $2 billion. Straight from the mouth of finance journalist Dan Carroll, "If you're looking for a hot stock to buy in the health care industry, few have garnered the attention that Intuitive Surgical has lately. The medical robotics maker has drawn in both bullish and bearish opinion aplenty as it pushes its surgical robots."[12]

Intuitive Surgical seems to be everywhere—on billboards, radio, and magazine ad pages—putting together a marketing campaign that *Mad Men*'s Don Draper would give the thumbs up to. The campaign features the ubiquitous loving couple, dancing or frolicking on the grass, the woman always gazing dreamily into her man's eyes. The subliminal message: have a da Vinci radical prostatectomy and before you know it you'll be dancing her into bed. The company's website features a plethora of upbeat information repeating the phrase "minimally invasive." On one of the many promotional videos, avuncular-sounding urologist Timothy Wilson, MD, says, "I tell men, it's simple; you have surgery, the prostate is out, you're recovered, you move on."[13]

But is it really that simple?

During a public education series sponsored by the cancer-patient-support organization, CancerCare, J. Francois Eid, MD, of Weill Cornell Medical College, briefly described some of the anatomical side effects men suffer after a radical prostatectomy. On the average, urologists perform between two to ten penile implants per year. Eid performs more than 300 implants per year, the highest number of anyone in the world.[14]

> There are some changes that occur to the penis after prostate cancer treatment and specifically that occurs after radical prostatectomy. We see shrinkage of the penis that occurs when the nerves are injured. We call that atrophy. There's also formation of scar tissue, lumps or bumps in the shaft of the penis. Some patients will have an hourglass deformity of the penile shaft or curvature of the penis. All of these physical alterations will not be noticeable by the patient if there is no sexual activity. So it's a reason to engage in sexual activity so that you can monitor to see what's happening. Why is it that important? Because if something is changing you want to consult your doctor so he can be proactive instead of waiting for the penis to shrink to a small size and be dissatisfied with the result.[15]

Your penis will shrink and have scar tissue, lumps and bumps, and perhaps an hourglass deformity. In his talk, Eid did note that even with a soft penis, a man might still have an orgasm. I wonder how many doctors have included this information in their informed discussions with their patients.

And according to CNBC reporter Herb Greenberg, a review of Intuitive Surgical internal documents along with interviews of surgeons, patients, lawyers, and ex-employees, found, among other things, a sharp rise in lawsuits and complaints about injuries, complications, and even deaths allegedly as a result of da Vinci surgery. It takes several hundred procedures to become proficient in robotic surgery. But surgeons can use the robot to operate on patients after just a few steps including an hour of online training, watching two videos, and seven hours operating on a pig! Moreover, the number of supervised cases varies by institution. Greenberg also cited Intuitive Surgical's high-pressure sales culture, motivated by "quotas" on surgical procedures that leads sales people to pressure surgeons to do more robotic surgeries.[16]

The da Vinci Surgical System is the only FDA-approved surgical robot on the market. Each unit costs close to $2 million dollars. Hospitals purchasing da Vinci robots must also agree to a $100,000 per year service contract. To CNBC reporter Greenberg's point about sales pressure, the heavy upfront price tag and expensive yearly service contract make it essential for hospitals to keep their robots busy with procedures. The pressing need to keep the da Vinci robots humming with patients might be one reason for a recent spate of reported injuries and adverse events (AEs), which include surgical burns to arteries, cut ureters (the tube that propels urine from the kidneys to the bladder), and sepsis (bacteria or their toxins in the blood or tissues). The FDA's MAUDE (Manufacturer and User Facility Device Experience) database shows that the number of AEs associated with the da Vinci Surgical System and its various instruments increased 34 percent from 2011 to 2012; during that period the number of da Vinci procedures increased by 26 percent. Consequently, Intuitive Surgical has been bombarded with litigation. At the writing of this book, Intuitive Surgical has been a defendant in at least 26 individual product-liability lawsuits filed by plaintiffs who contend that an equipment defect or inadequate training resulted in injury or death. In its quarterly report, Intuitive Surgical noted that the plaintiff's lawyers are "engaged in well-funded national advertising campaigns soliciting clients who have undergone da Vinci surgery and claim to have suffered an injury."[17]

Once again, the FDA has been behind the curve and patients suffer the consequences.

The growing number of AEs associated with robotic surgery should have caught the attention of the FDA sooner. In a survey letter sent to doctors who participate in the MAUDE product-safety network, the agency asked physicians to provide information about da Vinci robot performance and safety. Post-marketing efforts like this generally have little effect, as you'll see with the PSA test later. As for Intuitive Surgical, reports of robot-related injuries and FDA attention, so far, have not slowed the company's sales. In 2012 da Vinci robots were used in approximately 400,000 surgeries. That's triple the number of robotic surgeries done just four years ago. There are more than 1,400 hospitals in the United States and currently about one out of four has at least one da Vinci surgical robot. Not surprisingly, the most common da Vinci surgical procedure is for prostate cancer. In fact, about 85 percent of all radical prostatectomies in the United States are currently performed robotically.[18]

Most American men canvassed since the advent of robotic surgery say they chose robotic surgery because the doctors assured them of shorter recovery and fewer side effects. The term *minimally invasive* was usually the tipping point in their decision. The general feeling among men is that they'll be back to normal more quickly with robotic surgery than with standard open radical prostatectomy. The problem with that "feeling" is that the data do not support it!

But first a quick look at the procedure.

In traditional surgery to remove the prostate, called radical retropubic prostatectomy, the surgeon makes a long incision from the belly button to the pubic bone. In robotic surgery, called robotic-assisted laparoscopic radical prostatectomy, the surgeon sits at a video control panel apart from the operating table. After usual pre-op prep, the anesthetized man is placed on the operating table in what's called the Trendelenburg position; the table is tilted at a 45-degree angle so that the feet are above the head. The legs are parted and the robot is brought between the patient's feet. During the surgery, six punctures (less than an inch long) are made in the abdomen. Carbon dioxide is pumped (insufflation) into the abdomen to distend it, creating more room for the surgeon to operate. A thin tube with a camera on the end is placed into the puncture. The robot has four arms, one to hold the camera and three that have surgical instruments attached to their "hands." Using a foot pedal and a toggle, the lead surgeon controls the four robotic arms, placing them through four of the puncture incisions, while assistant surgeons work through the remaining two incisions. Using a scissorlike device and a foot-pedal-activated electrocautery clamp tool (using heat generated by high voltage to stop bleeding), the surgeon separates the prostate from the bladder and removes a portion of the sperm ducts and the seminal vesicles—a pair of glands situated on top of the prostate that secretes fluid that mixes with fluid from the prostate that ultimately becomes part of the semen. The prostate is then separated from the rectum, nerve sparing is performed in some men, and the urine channel at the tip of the prostate is divided. After the prostate and seminal vesicles are fully disconnected, the surgeon places them into a plastic bag while still inside the patient. The bag is removed by enlarging one of the incisions.

The bladder and urine channel are sutured together; a catheter is left in to help the healing process. The bagged specimens are sent to a pathology lab for analysis. The surgeon also might remove and send lymph nodes for pathological tests for cancer. A catheter is inserted through the penis and into the bladder to drain urine into a portable bag.

The whole procedure takes about three to four hours with da Vinci.

Because the prostate gland is located in a dense genitourinary area filled with nerve bundles and highly vascularized tissue, prostatectomy used to be a bloodier operation. An associate and friend, Dennis O'Hara, attested to that. O'Hara is a chapter founder and leader in the American Cancer Society (ACS) support program called Man-to-Man. He was diagnosed with prostate cancer in 1992, when he was 49 years old. "I had to give a pint of blood a week for four weeks prior to the operation. That's how bloody it was," he said, adding that for some unexplained motive the ACS terminated the Man-to-Man program nationwide. "I feel like they threw us under the bus," O'Hara fumed.[19] In retrospect, it would appear that the ACS, being a highly political organization, was distancing itself from pro-screening groups like Man-to-Man in the growing PSA debate.

Over the past decade, improved surgical techniques have made the procedure less bloody, which is one claim made by proponents of the da Vinci surgical system that might stand up to scrutiny. But the winning sales pitch for men rests on da Vinci's professed superiority over traditional surgery in preserving sexual function and urinary continence. And there is no clinical evidence to support the claims displayed on Intuitive Surgical's website in 23 video infomercials featuring media heavyweights from ABC's *Good Morning America* and CNN's "talking-head" doctor Sanjay Gupta, who said, "Studies show patients who undergo da Vinci prostatectomy may experience faster recovery from urinary incontinence following surgery . . . several studies show that patients who are potent prior to surgery have a high level of recovery of sexual function within a year following da Vinci surgery."[20]

However, results from a large-scale study published in 2009 tell a different story. The research team led by Jim Hu, MD, of Brigham and Women's Hospital in Boston, analyzed Medicare data for nearly 9,000 men who had prostatectomies between 2003 and 2007. Of those, 1,938 men had "minimally invasive surgery" (defined as either laparoscopic or robotic) and 6,899 had standard open prostatectomies. The men who had minimally invasive prostatectomies did leave the hospital one day sooner and tended to need fewer blood transfusions. However, there was no difference in cancer-recurrence rates between the two groups and in the most feared areas—urinary incontinence and impotence—the men who had minimally invasive surgery were more likely to report complications. Lead researcher Hu said, "The takeaway message is that men need to dig deeper than simply the message they're getting in planted stories from device makers or radio ads or billboards."[21]

More recently, a paper published in 2012 in the *Journal of Clinical Oncology* (*JCO*) compared the severity of side effects between traditional open radical prostatectomy and robotic prostatectomy. The paper concluded: "Risks of problems with incontinence and sexual function are high after both procedures. Medicare-age men should not expect fewer adverse effects following robotic prostatectomy."[22] The nationally regarded authors of the *JCO* study, Drs. Michael Barry and Floyd Fowler Jr., are with the Foundation for Informed Medical Decision Making. This is a robust organization that does valuable bipartisan health-policy research, offering workable solutions to thorny issues affecting our health care system. A line from the foundation's mission statement sums up much of the trepidation the FDA Advisory Panel voiced in 1993 about the use of routine PSA screening of healthy men: "We believe that the only way to ensure high quality medical decisions are being made is for a fully informed patient to participate in a shared decision making process with their health care provider."[23] Ironically, the foregoing has recently been adopted by the American Urological Association (AUA) in its new 2013 guidelines for PSA screening.[24]

But prior to the new AUA guidelines, "shared decision making" was not part of the PSA story. We know that for 30-plus years, men of a certain age were—and still are—given a PSA test as part of their yearly physical exam. When it comes to making treatment decisions, most men do not know the clinical risks involved or all the possible results and outcomes of treatments. The availability of technology shouldn't give people the license to use it, especially when there's no proof of its benefit. Our medical history is full of examples of hastily contrived evidence leading to widespread deployment of procedures with distressing consequences for patients.

You've just read about $200 million proton-beam centers being built largely on the projected income from prostate cancer. Yet there's little to no evidence that proton therapy is better than a far less costly route. Then we have the extravagant $2 million da Vinci robot, which also uses prostate cancer as its piggy bank and with insufficient scientific evidence to support the claims of less impotence and better urinary control. Evidence aside, slick advertising replete with glowing testimonials and frolicking couples has certainly helped Intuitive Surgical penetrate the prostate market.

The company slogan might just as well read: "Robots Do It Better!"

But not so fast. What happens if multiple lawsuits roll out and patients who have had da Vinci robotic surgery start coming out of the woodwork, claiming they were misled about the robot's side-effect benefits and safety? Suppose additional follow-up studies confirm that da Vinci is no more effective than traditional laparoscopy (just much more costly), and the procedure is susceptible to dangerous human and technical errors? Remember, Intuitive Surgical has only one product: da Vinci. And it is the only FDA-approved robotic system for soft-tissue surgery. In effect, they have a monopoly on robotic prostatectomies. But a flood of future lawsuits, negative press, and damning studies could expose da Vinci as a high-priced technology that doesn't live up to the hype. If that happens, the more than 1,400 hospitals that have laid out $2 million per da Vinci system and have committed themselves to a $100,000 per year service contract are stuck with an overpriced machine that can't pay for itself.

This could be a medical and financial disaster in the making. Sadly, it was preventable. The FDA approved the da Vinci system based on Intuitive Surgical's study data, comparing 113 patients who had da Vinci surgery to 132 patients who underwent traditional laparoscopy—the results were comparable; *neither* group showed an advantage.[25] More important, the surgery involved in the study was gall bladder removal, a simple surgery compared to the incredibly complex set of challenges involved in a radical prostatectomy. It is worth repeating: the FDA approved this robotic surgical system that is now performing hundreds of thousands of radical prostatectomies on the strength of 113 gallbladder procedures!

This serves as yet another example of how our regulatory system approves drugs and devices without having sufficient evidence of their safety and effectiveness, bowing to the will of industry instead of being a solid gatekeeper for American health care.

But health care consumers need not be health care zombies.

Why do we so readily accept the promotional carpet bombing (or carpetbagging) by drug and device companies touting their latest technology or drug? One explanation is that—even in the absence of evidence—certain drugs and technologies make sense to us. In effect, their supposed utility wins us over. For example, it seems plausible that the highly controlled particle beam delivered to prostate cancer in a spaceship-sized proton-beam facility must be better than the less accurate "traditional" (read "old") radiation treatment. After absorbing the seductive sales pitch, health care consumers begin to view traditional radiation like a shotgun spray compared with proton beam's sniper-bullet accuracy. Likewise, potential patients naturally assume robotic surgery is safer than "old-style" open surgery. Think of the visual image: a gleaming high-tech machine hooked to computers versus a bloody-handed human wielding a gleaming knife.

Proton-beam therapy and da Vinci robotic surgery are but two examples in which proponents of routine PSA screening have hardened their position in the face of overwhelming data showing that screening does far more harm than good. But again, as radiation oncologist Zietman bluntly stated, "This is a high-stakes game. Without prostate cancers to treat, they [proton beam centers and the Da Vinci Surgical System] will fail." The medical industry spends an inordinate amount of money to create innovative products, but it also spends an equal amount of its funds to systematically change the behavior of consumers and doctors to ensure that their products are purchased.[26] As you've seen with proton beam centers and da Vinci robots, it's a big-bucks cycle of marketing trumping evidence.

I'll further explore the financial incentives driving the prostate cancer industry, but the point about our culture's readiness to accept the rapid diffusion of the newest drug or medical device—before solid evidence of safety and effectiveness—needs a bit more discussion. A 2008 paper by Bruce Leff and Thomas Finucane in the *Journal of the American Medical Association* makes the case that a phenomenon the authors call "gizmo idolatry" has changed the practice of medicine. According to the authors,

> The word "gizmo" refers to a mechanical device or procedure for which the clinical benefit in a specific clinical context is not clearly established, and "gizmo idolatry" refers to the general implicit conviction that a more technological approach is intrinsically better than one that is less technological unless, or perhaps even if, there is strong evidence to the contrary.[27]

Proton beam therapy and da Vinci robotic surgery certainly fall into the gizmo idolatry bucket, since these gizmos have saturated the prostate cancer market despite insufficient evidence of superior effectiveness over less expensive counterparts. A market-driven society with an aging population, such as ours, is a textbook environment for entrepreneur-minded doctors and scientists to promote new medical technologies and drugs. The potential profits are irresistible. Big Oil is a popular punching bag for DC politicians looking for an easy fat cat to pillory; however, Big Oil's estimated profit margin of 8.3 percent pales in comparison to Big Pharma's average 15.4 percent profit. There's another important distinction beyond profit: oil does what it purports to do—it keeps our homes warm and our cars and trucks on the road. But as numerous studies have shown, many of the expensive drugs pumping up the pharmaceutical industry's bottom line are ineffective—they simply don't fulfill their intended medical purpose.[28]

The drug and device industries, in their tireless self-promotion efforts, adroitly maneuver all the players into their high-rolling game of science for sale. Richard Horton, editor of the internationally regarded medical journal *The Lancet,* gives a terse appraisal of how far we've strayed from the fundamental responsibility of rigorous science reporting, an essential check and balance. "Journals have devolved into information laundering operations for the pharmaceutical industry."[29] And, as we've seen with the PSA test, the medical-device industry, too.

LET'S TAKE A BRIEF SIDE TRIP off the main PSA highway, down a dark road to our not-so-distant medical past. It's a road that vividly exposes how susceptible we are to many forms of medical idolatry. And while not PSA-based, there are some parallels in this story worth noting. They speak to the failure of the underlying structure that is supposed to protect people from profit- and ego-driven predators and assure the robust functioning of the health care market. It's a fine line that's far too easy to blur.

Listening to Howard Dully talk is like hearing a drowsy actor doing a movie voice-over. There's an "I'm here but not really" feel to the conversation. "I've always felt different, wondered if something was missing from my soul," said Dully.[30] At 56, he's finally coming to a place in his life that is absolved from the tug of past secrets which have kept him wondering why he feels the way he does. When Dully was 12 years old, his stepmother, an unbalanced woman, brought him to a hospital to have a lobotomy. Her reason was that Howard was a troublesome boy. That was enough evidence for Dr. Walter Freeman. He took the young boy into a room, administered four rounds of electroshock treatment to knock him senseless, then he pushed an icepick-like instrument underneath the boy's orbital bone just above the eyeball. In a quick scrambling motion, Freeman severed the tissue in the prefrontal lobes of Dully's brain. The procedure took about ten minutes.

Nobody was there to stand up for the young boy and demand to see the scientific evidence proving that this crude procedure even approached the safe and effective threshold. But by then, Freeman was a famous neuropsychiatrist, doing up to 20 lobotomies a day. He was a celebrity of sorts and no one dared question him.

The theoretical underpinnings for psychosurgery began in Europe in the early twentieth century during a time of wild and unfettered experimentation. A woman with postpartum depression could be treated in any number of ways, such as convulsive therapy, malarial therapy, insulin shock treatment, or deep sleep therapy (essentially being put into a drug-induced coma). Freeman became fascinated by the aggressive procedures coming out of Europe, most notably from the Portuguese neurologist Egas Moniz, an early and enthusiastic proponent of the lobotomy. Moniz later became a mentor and idol for Freeman. In 1949 Moniz won the Noble Prize in physiology and medicine for his discovery of the "therapeutic value of leucotomy [lobotomy] in certain psychoses." He theorized that the cure for certain mental illnesses was an assault on the brain.

After almost ten years of performing prefrontal lobotomies—a labor-intensive procedure that entails drilling holes in the skull—Freeman, a reductionist at heart, heard of an Italian doctor named Amarro Fiamberti who performed lobotomies through the patient's eye sockets. The transorbital approach was a perfect fit for the hard-charging Freeman, allowing him to perform lobotomies in hallways, if necessary, so overcrowded and understaffed were state mental institutions. Forever the showman, Freeman crisscrossed the country—in his personal van he dubbed the lobotomobile—doing icepick surgeries and playing to the crowds of young interns and nurses.

His most famous lobotomy was performed on John F. Kennedy's sister, Rosemary Kennedy, an emotionally frail woman with an unsuitably low IQ and a habit of acting out, which proved an embarrassment for the family's patriarch, bootlegger, and kingmaker, Joseph P. Kennedy. When Rosemary was 23, on the suggestion of the family's doctor, Kennedy took his free-spirited daughter to see Freeman and his then-partner Dr. James W. Watts. This was in 1941, when Freeman was still performing prefrontal lobotomies, done through incisions at the top of the skull. Freeman's later fervent transition to the less laborious icepick technique would leave Watts squeamish, ending their relationship.

Here's a brief description of Rosemary Kennedy's lobotomy. According to Watts, the instrument they used looked like a butter knife. After drilling holes in her head and making incisions, he swung the blade up and down to cut brain tissue. Watts explained that when the instrument was inside her skull, he began to swing it back and forth as Freeman asked Rosemary to recite the Lord's Prayer or sing "God Bless America" or count backwards. They used her answers to estimate how deeply to cut into the brain. When she became incoherent, they stopped.[31] The lobotomy left the 23-year-old woman permanently incapacitated. For the better part of her remaining life, Rosemary Kennedy lived in a cottage on the grounds of St. Coletta School for Exceptional Children. Her father never visited her; she died of natural causes in 2005.

Although skeptics in the medical community were growing uneasy about Freeman's zeal for the icepick lobotomy, he was an undeterred self-promoter and his public bravado and force of personality only accelerated the procedure's use. Wolfhard Baumgartel, a staff physician at the Athens State Hospital in Ohio, was present during a series of Freeman's lobotomies. He described himself at the time a "green beginner who hardly spoke any English, and he [Freeman] was a big shot." Baumgartel recalls that on one particular day

Freeman did about 20 lobotomies, never once leaving the operating room. "The patient went out, the next patient was ready to come in, had his procedure done, went out again, and then the next patient came in," said Baumgartel, as he described the macabre assembly line.[32]

Baumgartel recalled Freeman as being oddly relaxed and calm while inserting the icepick through the orbital bone and into the person's brain. "He had an extremely self-confident personality. He wanted to prove he was right. He was convinced he was right. But I thought to myself, how can a man be so relaxed just going blindly into a person's brain? But I had no authority to tell him to stop!" Baumgartel added that after the procedure there seemed to be some intangible thing missing in the person. "Just take all your emotion away and what's left?"

The answer to Baumgartel's rhetorical question is that the affected area in Freeman's procedures is the prefrontal lobe of the cerebral cortex, which in varying degrees controls decisions, creativity, movement, reasoning, memory, and sexual behavior. The damage depended on the vigor of Freeman's icepick. Its results could be subtle or vegetative.

In 1967 Freeman performed his last icepick lobotomy on a longtime patient named Helen Mortensen. He had lobotomized her twice before. She died from a brain hemorrhage following the third procedure. After Mortensen's death, Freeman was finally banned from doing lobotomies, but by then 40,000 to 50,000 people had already been lobotomized in the United States alone.

To a reader, the natural question would be: Is Dr. Richard J. Ablin comparing an icepick lobotomy to a radical prostatectomy? The answer, of course, is no. Freeman's lobotomies had all the scientific finesse and exactness of a blindfolded short-order cook scrambling eggs. But his carte blanche ravaging of human brains—about 3,500—without supporting evidence is worth noting within this book's context since it happened a stone's throw back in our history. In fact, Freeman performed his last icepick lobotomy in 1967, the same year that Dr. Christian Bernard performed the world's first heart transplant—an evidence-based procedure that transformed medicine.

So one must ask, why, at a contemporaneous time of great medical advances, was an egomaniacal butcher like Freeman allowed to crisscross the country jamming an ice pick into people's brains—a middle-aged housewife with postpartum depression, for instance, or a 12-year-old whose unbalanced stepmother wanted an easy-to-control zombie instead of a roughhousing boy? Where was the American Medical Association? Where were the outraged speeches on the floor of the Senate? Where were the patient advocates? Where was the evidence?

Freeman didn't need evidence; he had the crowd behind him.

IN 1993 ECONOMISTS CALCULATED that routine PSA screening of men 50 years and older, along with the subsequent tests and procedures, costs our health care system about $28 billion per year.[33] There are a lot of moving parts in determining costs on such a massive scale; however, no matter how you slice and dice the numbers, the economic drain from routine PSA screening is staggering. And it all begins with a test that costs about $80. But before we drill deeper into those numbers, let's take a brief overview of where the problem begins: our gluttonous, passive-aggressive, fee-for-service health care system that enables widespread exploitation of its finite resources.

We are consistently told a convenient and self-serving untruth that the United States has the best health care system in the world. It's true that we have the most expensive health care system, nearly double the per capita spending of Norway and Sweden, the next highest-spending countries in the Organization for Economic Cooperation and Development. Roughed out, we spend about $8,000 per person compared with Norway's $4,000 per person. Most health care analysts agree that we're not getting our money's worth. For decades, studies have fingered the same culprits: health services are wasted, repeated, overdone, and harmful, which results in more treatments—the quintessential vicious cycle of overutilization of services.

There are numerous metrics used to gauge the quality of health care. In 2000 the World Health Organization (WHO) ranked the health systems of its 191 member states; the United States was ranked a dismally low 38th in the world. WHO used a series of performance indicators to assess the overall level and availability of health care and the responsiveness and financing of health care services. For instance, in the measure looking at life expectancy from birth, we rank 50th in the world. The United States also ranks fairly low in infant mortality rates, about 34th in the world. Mortality statistics have shock value but they don't give a clear picture of the complexities of our system, which, in many ways, is still the envy of the world.

For example, US life expectancy figures are held down by factors that the health care system has no direct control over, such as homicides, motor vehicle deaths, and poor diet and lack of exercise. Plus it's statistically irrational to compare small, rather homogeneous countries like Norway—whose population is about the same as that of the state of Louisiana—to a vast country like the United States, which has dramatic socioeconomic variations across multiple racial and ethnic groups. Our health care problems are, in part, disparities in access to care (perhaps no better exemplified than by African Americans), rather than lack of having quality care.

Another significant flaw is that, unlike most European countries, our system does not evaluate drugs and devices for their cost-effectiveness (the minimal expenditure of dollars, time, and other elements necessary to achieve the health care result deemed necessary and appropriate.). By law, Medicare must pay for any drug that is approved by the FDA, no matter how costly, even when there's another equally effective and less expensive drug. Studies show that in the lucrative cancer-drug market, many oncologists base their treatment decisions on which drug provides their practice with the most profit. To that point, oncologists treating lung cancer have eight different chemotherapy drugs to choose from; all have the same relative benefit to the patient. The cheapest of these is paclitaxel, which costs Medicare about $1,322 per month. The most expensive is pemetrexed, which costs more than $7,000 per month—almost seven times as much. If you're comparing the price of a filet mignon to a hot dog, then yes, you get what you pay for. But why spend so much more on a drug that isn't much better than its least expensive counterpart?

There's a decidedly more dramatic example of how our system incentivizes the "doctor-greed gene." Men with advanced prostate cancer face a grim prognosis. (I'll discuss this in more detail a bit down the road.) Oncologists, until approximately the past two to three years had relatively few therapeutic options, especially in men with castration-resistant prostate cancer, which means that they don't respond to drugs that suppress the hormones that accelerate the growth of prostate cancer. ("Castration" in this context refers to chemical castration rather than surgical removal of the testicles.) These men are at the end of their clinical rope, with few treatment options. One option is an immunotherapy called Provenge, which costs a mind-numbing $93,000 for the three infusion treatments. (Immunotherapies are designed to boost the ability of the body's immune system to destroy cancer cells.) Another option is the standard-of-care generic drug docetaxel, which costs Medicare a meager $585 per month. Provenge was approved because it purportedly extends the life of these men by about four months.

Since the bulk of medical oncologists' revenue comes from the drugs they prescribe, it's not difficult to conclude that many doctors are simply taking advantage of what the system is offering.[34]

Health policy expert Peter Bach, MD, simplifies this complicated issue. His use of cancer drugs to illustrate waste and abuse can be generalized across most sectors of the health care market.

The drug manufacturers in the United States essentially have no downward pressure on the cost of cancer drugs. They can choose to charge whatever they like. There's been this long period where manufacturers are getting increasingly bold in terms of the prices they're willing to charge. One of them comes on the market with a drug with a high price, and no one flinches. Then the next one has no hesitation to charge a similar price. So we see this almost lock-step progression in the rise of the cost of cancer drugs and no check on that.[35]

If the drugs worked, the high cost could be partially justified. But most don't. Most of the people reading this book will still manage to navigate their way through the health care system without really needing to think about cost-effectiveness or sticker-shock-priced drugs that have little value. But it can't be pleasant to think that if this trend of reckless profiteering isn't addressed in the near future, our country's health care system will go over the cliff. It's unthinkable. But it will happen.

THE PURPOSE OF THAT BRIEF DISCUSSION on perverse incentives driving up our health care spending was not to disparage the health care system—even though constructive criticism is often met with reflexive anger by those who are milking it dry—but rather to add more context to my central point that money, power, and cronyism within the big medicine industry have hijacked the PSA test and created a national health care disaster. I've already exposed some of the central players and the strategies employed to morph a simple blood test into a moneymaking juggernaut. The question that needs to be asked over and over is: What effect does the behavior I'm describing have on you, the innocent health care consumer? In a short while you'll meet a man who has made countless millions in the prostate cancer industry.

Cost in health care, as in any consumer product or service, is based on value, which in health care is defined as outcomes relative to costs. It's a lot easier to assess value in a product like an automobile than it is in health care, simply because it's easier to gauge value in a car—if it starts on the first turn of the key, drives well, and looks good, we tend to think it has its advertised value. Our bodies, on the other hand, are fragile and mysterious. That's why we trust doctors to use the right tools, treatments, and drugs to keep us healthy, especially as we age.

As I've argued from the opening pages, the test does not do what it purports to do—detect cancer. Further, the survival studies I've referenced show that men diagnosed with prostate cancer who had radical prostatectomies on average lived no longer than men who opted out of treatment. Remember Dr. William J. Catalona's presentation to the FDA advisory panel on behalf of Hybritech? Even he, the high priest of the radical prostatectomy, admitted there was no evidence that radical prostatectomies extended men's lives. Then there's the test itself. As I mentioned, there are two standard ways to calibrate the test: the WHO way and the Hybritech way. Not surprisingly, Catalona urges using the Hybritech way. Making matters even more confusing is a report by the Mayo Clinic finding that in the approximate field of 16 different PSA test models, there is a 5 to 40 percent variance in the PSA number.[36] In that mix of testing variables, the question to biopsy or not to biopsy is like playing PSA roulette.

Why is the public not aware of these wild disparities in PSA testing results? Apply this scenario to the auto industry. Imagine that the test that manufacturers used to verify the safety of brakes was calibrated with the same haphazard disregard for accuracy. Public advocates would be up in arms. There would be massive recalls from GM and Ford and congressional hearings full of windy outcry.

EARLY WARNING

On January 17, 1960, President Dwight Eisenhower gave the country an ominous warning about a threat to our democratic government: "the military-industrial complex." He worried, and rightfully so, that unchecked alliances between self-serving entities would create a greed-driven monopoly of sorts, debasing the central purpose of the military—protecting the country. Eisenhower said, "In the councils of government, we must guard against the acquisition of unwarranted influence, whether sought or unsought, by the military-industrial complex. The potential for the disastrous rise of misplaced power exists, and will persist."[37]

Eisenhower's stark warning is threaded into the fabric of this book; of course, the threat here is from the medical-industrial complex. We saw how Dr. Anthony Zietman warned about the medical arms race that was being fueled by prostate cancer. We looked at $200 million proton-beam centers and $2 million robots. A torrential river of money runs through the prostate cancer industry; some of its tributaries are streams, but they all feed into the central ocean of green water. As PSA testing slowly begins to lose its grip, the stakeholders become alarmed. Without PSA, they fail.

Let's wade down a few streams.

Well-to-do California urologist Douglas O. Chinn, MD, a partner with his brother in Chinn & Chinn Urology Associates, holds several patents in prostate cancer-related treatments. Chinn is also a huge proponent of PSA screening. One treatment he proselytizes for is HIFU (high-intensity-focused ultrasound). The theory behind HIFU is that high-intensity, focused sonic energy can be used to locally heat and destroy cancerous tissue. The FDA has not approved the procedure; it remains at the investigation stage in the United States and is being studied in clinical trials.

Hypothetically—because there is no residual accumulation of data as in radiation—an infinite number of HIFU treatments can be given, which makes solid business sense. Chinn gives a very elegant PowerPoint presentation promoting HIFU.[38] He himself is an elegant and polished spokesperson for treatments like HIFU. There's one problem, one that keeps recurring in this story: there are scant data supporting HIFU's clinical value. Yet prostate cancer patients make this incredible leap of faith when they walk into Chinn's office.

Another leap-of-faith example is urologist Ronald Wheeler, MD, medical director at the Diagnostics Center for Disease, Sarasota, Florida, in association with PanAm HIFU. He treats prostate cancer patients with HIFU in well-heeled sections of Cancun and London. Wheeler boasts, "Cancun offers spectacular 'medical tourism' as well as five-star hospital facilities."[39]

Chinn, an ardent supporter of PSA screening, voiced his opinion in a recent article titled "Prostate Cancer, To Screen or Not to

Screen: What a Stupid Question or How the USPSTF Got It All Wrong." A sentence in the article jumped out at me when I read it. It demonstrates just how out of touch the urology community is with the men they treat. While bashing the US Preventive Services Task Force's recommendation against routine PSA screening, Chinn said, "the underlying theme of the Task / Force is that the *very small risks* of biopsy and the *small side effect risks* of cancer treatment far outweighs the side effects of prostate cancer [emphasis added]."[40]

Categorizing impotence and incontinence as *small* strikes a profoundly insensitive chord to men, one that rings throughout the industry. How else could they advise men to have procedures that the straight-talking urologist Burt Vorstman says may "[leave] a man limp and leaking"?

Vorstman believes that the radical surgical/robotic treatment option has been the major factor for the increased incidence of impotence and incontinence worldwide. "Physicians would do well to consider the Hippocrates affirmation: As to diseases, make a habit of two things—to help, or at least, to do no harm. Men who choose these treatments without reviewing an alternative are playing Russian roulette with their quality-of-life prospects following the surgery," Vorstman told me during an interview.[41] He assails most invasive urologic procedures as "an attack on manhood." Strong words, but not an angry tirade from an outsider with an ax to grind; it's a frank assessment from a urologist on the front lines of cancer care who has seen the damage done to men.

LIMP AND LEAKING

Let's get back to money and some of the industries that profit off the effects Chinn alluded to. The big two side effects—incontinence and impotence—have fueled cottage medical industries. True, these industries are tiny compared to proton-beam centers, surgical robots, and drugs, but they still are moneymaking machines. Penile implants, erectile dysfunction drugs and devices, urinary cuffs, diapers, catheters—the list goes on.

I'll start with incontinence, which is the involuntary leakage of urine. Here's an excerpt from an article in the highly regarded medical journal *Advances in Urology:*

> Post prostatectomy incontinence can have devastating effects on the quality of life of patients treated for prostate cancer and may result in considerable psychological morbidity. Post prostatectomy incontinence itself can be difficult to treat, and concomitant bladder neck contracture [shortening of] presents an even more challenging clinical problem.[42]

Urinary incontinence can have a profoundly negative impact on a man's life. Over the years I've received literally thousands of e-mails from men who are at various points in the prostate cancer gamut. To put a face on incontinence, I've amalgamated a composite man from those e-mails, a man who recently had his prostate removed and is now dealing with incontinence. This "case study" represents the middle ground of postsurgery incontinence—a slightly worse-than-average problem, but nowhere near the worst-case scenario. Although a composite, this man is a flesh-and-blood reality of post-prostatectomy incontinence. Scott is a 55-year-old self-employed carpenter who is married and has two sons. During his yearly physical, his primary doctor detected that his PSA was 4.3. Without any discussion other than the usual, "it's probably nothing, but let's make sure," Scott was biopsied; the biopsy came back positive for prostate cancer. Urged by his wife and that feeling of mortality being compressed into a millisecond, Scott had a radical prostatectomy. By all accounts, the surgery was successful. The surgeon gave a thumbs up, everything was clear. (As a side note, there is no way that a surgeon can back up the post-op claims of "we got it all.")

Scott was incontinent immediately after surgery, but his doctor assured him that it would resolve within a few weeks. But it didn't. During each follow-up visit, Scott was reassured that the "problem" would get better. The weeks turned to months. Scott finally stopped seeing the surgeon. He had no problem at night, but when he rolled from bed in the morning his penis would leak profusely. He was using high-absorbency pads (diapers) that tied around his hips. He tried doing Kegel exercises—repetitively contracting and releasing muscles of the pelvic floor, which stretch from the anus to the urinary sphincter, the muscle that maintains constriction of an orifice, in this case the opening between the bladder and the ureter. But Kegels didn't help. He was going through about five to six absorbent pads a day. Imagine a working man having to change his pad continually throughout the day. Scott was in trouble. At 55, he was an active person who played golf and sports with his kids. Now he couldn't—any stress forced urine from his bladder. A piece of his life was gone. And it was embarrassing. That's the way he put it. Embarrassing. He'd gone from feeling intensely alive to this.

Sex was the furthest thing from his mind at this point. He was still impotent from the prostatectomy, but he was hopeful that in time he would regain enough potency to attempt having sex with his wife. The incontinency was also a roadblock to sex. (Urine can leak during sex.) Think of trying to become sexually intimate while wearing a diaper. Vorstman's "limp and leaking" phrase brutally described Scott's feeling of falling away.

A year into the ordeal Scott was still incontinent and growing desperate. Through an acquaintance, he heard about an incontinence-relief procedure called bulbourethral sling surgery. He consulted another surgeon who had performed many successful sling surgeries. Scott had the surgery; the recovery was even tougher than the radical prostatectomy. Briefly, the surgeon makes an incision between the scrotum and the rectum and installs a supportive sling under and around the urethra, anchoring it on each side of the pelvic bone. Theoretically, by placing pressure on the urethra, the sling helps retain urine while the bladder fills. The operation was physically and mentally taxing. Then disaster struck—the sling procedure didn't work. Scott couldn't control his bladder. He was devastated.

Six months later Scott came across another possible solution, an artificial sphincter. He met with a surgeon and decided to try it. In the procedure, the surgeon inserts a small pump into the scrotum, which is attached to a sphincter cuff and a small balloon located near the belly button. When Scott feels the need to urinate, he goes to the bathroom and squeezes the pump in his scrotum with one hand. By pressing the pump, it deflates the cuff, and pressure comes off the urethra, allowing him to urinate. In about 40 seconds, the balloon fills back up. If Scott feels he hasn't voided completely, he does the squeeze procedure again. The artificial sphincter worked, giving Scott about 90 percent bladder control. He still uses light absorbent pads to catch occasional drips. Despite having a three-piece device inserted into his body, Scott can now lead a normal life. Next, he'll begin dealing with his erectile dysfunction.

Before drilling into more cost issues, it's important that every health care consumer be aware of the potential dangers involved in medical procedures. Do some research and question your doctor. And be armed with credible data. In Scott's situation, having an artificial urinary sphincter was his best bet to regain continence. He was on the edge of the cliff. But whenever you have a foreign device surgically implanted in your body there are inherent risks, such as infection or device failure. You don't want to fall into the category of patients whose vast clinical knowledge is acquired through a cycle of misadventures.

I previously mentioned the FDA's MAUDE site. It's where AEs are voluntarily reported and it's open to the public. Scott had a relatively good experience with his artificial sphincter surgery. But there are many device makers that produce artificial sphincters and not all of them are the same quality. Then there's the variability of the surgeon's skill. At the MAUDE site, just punch in the key words *artificial sphincter* and the pages pop up. As of the writing of this book there were about 2,500 pages, each page containing ten reports. This doesn't include the FDA's archive and only voluntary reports. Each of the 25,000 or so reported medical errors on MAUDE was an unnecessary expense that set in motion more procedures and in many cases lawsuits. Below are two verbatim MAUDE report descriptions of malfunctions that occurred in the kind of device Scott had implanted.

Event Date: 01/21/2010

Event Type: Malfunction

Event Description: Failure of artificial cuff. Pinhole leak was found in cuff, which required replacement of hydraulic fluid.[43]

Event Date: 01/21/2010

Event Type: Malfunction

Event Description: During surgery, a control pump for an artificial sphincter failed to operate correctly at the time of implantation. The back up pump was opened to use, but it also failed to operate correctly. The other components were implanted successfully. The patient will be brought back at a later time as an outpatient to have the pump implanted.[44]

I would not describe what Scott endured as a "small side effect" of prostate cancer treatment. He went through hell and his journey was costly—besides the Goliath-like expenditures such as proton beam centers and robotic surgery, the prostate industry nickels and dimes the system to death.

Since his PSA test, Scott racked up a substantial medical bill. The biopsy cost about $2,000; the radical prostatectomy ran upward of $30,000. Plus, he had two post-op procedures for incontinence. The unsuccessful bulbourethral sling surgery cost several thousand dollars and the subsequent artificial sphincter procedure cost many times more; the device itself without surgical billing runs upward of $8,000. These are unavoidable downstream costs in the aftermath of radical prostatectomy. Besides big-ticket surgical procedures, multiple ancillary costs, such as diapers, are overlooked in prostate cancer's massive money pit. Men, like Scott, who have prostatectomies need absorbent pads to catch and deodorize persistently leaking urine, which opens the market for the Kimberly-Clark Corporation, an American personal care company that produces mostly paper-based consumer products. The company is listed in the Fortune 500. Business is booming, in part because Kimberly-Clark leverages every market opportunity by rolling out celebrities to pitch their products. The company website uses manly men to hawk their male incontinence-product line.[45] The headline "Guard Your Manhood with Depend Guards and Shields" features a video with macho ex–pro-football player Tony "The Goose" Siragusa. Tony is there to lead you through a Depend training session. Mounted on the wall behind big Tony is a huge moose head. A pair of boxing gloves dangles nearby. This is no place for wimps. Tony makes that clear from the get-go. "Leaks should never get in the way of doing your thing—you just need to get the right plan in place. If you're not using Depend guards or shields, you're probably not getting the right protection." Tony picks up a basket full of feminine hygiene products and barks, "See this. This is for girls, not for you!" and tosses the sissified items across the room.

Men like Scott can easily go through eight to ten Depend diapers a day, at about $1 a piece, depending on the particular product. That's at least $4,000 a year.

Kimberly-Clark also has an altruistic side.

In 2009 Kimberly-Clark's Depend brand launched the "The Depend Campaign to End Prostate Cancer."[46] According to the company, it's a four-month campaign in celebration of Men's Health Month that culminates with National Prostate Cancer Awareness Month, which "engages a star-studded lineup of sports legends as campaign ambassadors and awareness advocates." One legend, Hall of Fame quarterback Jim Kelly, lends his brand name to a video in which he describes his most recent PSA test, offering commentary.

A company spokesperson notes that a portion of the proceeds from the purchase of each package of Depend underwear or guards will be donated to ZERO—The Project to End Prostate Cancer, purportedly to help fund education and research. First off, the word *education* is interchangeable with *PSA*. Kimberly-Clark is in this for the buck. But after all the years of profits and fundraising and free PSA tests, it is fair to ask representatives from ZERO exactly how their efforts have helped the overall effort to find a cure for prostate cancer. Mark Cammarota, marketing director for Kimberly-Clark, noted that about 4 million men in the United States are currently managing some form of incontinence, "many of whom are doing so as a result of a prostate-related health issue."[47]

Prostate cancer-treatment-related incontinence is a huge business. The American market for disposable incontinence garments has exploded in recent years, with estimated annual sales of $1.32 billion in 2011, compared with $557 million in 1997. That's an increase of 137 percent. Depend is the leading brand, with a 30.8 percent market share. According to the Kantar Media unit of WPP (a world leader in marketing communications), Depend spent $13.1 million on advertising in 2011, compared with $10.2 million in 2010.[48]

THE ED COTTAGE INDUSTRY

Now let's move to another prostate cancer cottage industry: erectile dysfunction (ED).

An erection begins in the brain. It sounds easy, but sexual arousal is a complex mental, hormonal, and physical process that, in part, remains a mystery. To better understand this process, researchers used functional MRI, an imaging procedure that measures brain activity by detecting associated changes in blood flow. They found a complex neural circuit was involved in human males during sexual arousal with a specific correlation between erection and activations in anterior cingulate, insula, amygdala, and hypothalamus regions of the brain.[49] In short, the penile erection process emerges in the part of the brain that stores our most primitive responses.

A penile erection is central to the consciousness of being a man. First and foremost, the physiologic purpose of an erection is to penetrate the female vagina and ejaculate sperm to fertilize an egg resulting in the development of the fetus and the subsequent birth of another human being. A flaccid penis falls short in continuing the human species. Throughout the ages, male virility has been the dramatic counterpoint to potent female sexual power. Male history is tied to the erection: ancient phallic images painted on cave walls, carved in wood, sculpted in marble, and scratched as graffiti art on subway cars.

The mythological fertility god, Priapus, with his absurdly over-sized, permanent erection gives his name to the eponymous medical condition priapism, in which the erect penis does not return to its flaccid state, despite the absence of both physical and psychological stimulation, within four hours—the much heard four-hour warning in Viagra commercials. The universally shared sexual performance angst among men helps drive the erectile prostate cancer ED busi-ness. Viagra, Pfizer's $1 billion-a-year blockbuster drug is known to every man in the United States. One pill costs $15 to $22, which can be quite costly. Viagra, or similar products, is the first-line treatment for ED following prostatectomy or radiation therapy.[50] Second-line treatment is usually penile injections, which I'll discuss in a later chapter. The last resort on the ED treatment pyramid is a surgical procedure, the penile implant.

Being able to attain and sustain a penetrable erection is essential for male health. As obsessively important as it is to men, most know more about a carburetor than about their penis and the erection pro-cess. The penis contains three-cylinder-shaped masses of erectile tis-sue, two corpora cavernosa, which lie side by side and above a third mass, the corpus spongiosum urethra. The urethra is the channel through which urine and sperm flow. The shaft is the longest part of the penis. The head (glans penis) is located at the end of the shaft. The opening at the tip of the head is called the meatus, where urine and semen are discharged. Erectile tissue contains blood vessels, two main arteries, and nerves.

When a man gets sexually aroused, physical and mental stimula-tion cause nerves in the brain to send chemical messages telling the penile blood vessels to relax so that blood can flow freely into the penis. First, the penis increases in length and girth as high pressure traps the blood within both corpora cavernosa, allowing further expansion and a sustainable erection. The firmness of the erection depends on maintaining high blood pressure in the cavernous bod-ies. It's called vasocongestion, which is simply the swelling of tissues caused by increased vascular blood and localized blood pressure. It's the process that also causes menstrual cramps in women.

Healthy veins and undisturbed nerves are instrumental to achieving an erection. This is where the radical prostatectomy does its damage. Nerves that control erections pass across and adhere fully to the prostate gland. Separating this nerve bundle has been compared to peeling wet tissue paper from a surface. No matter how skilled the surgeon is, there is always a certain amount of nerve damage during a radical prostatectomy, resulting in various degrees and duration of impotence.

In cases when the nerve damage and other physiologic issues result in permanent impotence, the last resort for many men is a penile implant. It's a major decision to have a medical device surgically implanted in a very delicate body part, made more difficult by two possible downsides: a risk of infection and a risk that the device won't work. The surgery is fairly straightforward, taking about 40 minutes or so. While the man is under general anesthesia, a Foley catheter is inserted through the penis and the bladder is emptied. An incision is made across the top of the scrotum at the base of the penis.

There are two main types of implants: malleable and hydraulic inflatable prostheses. Malleable implants usually consist of a pair of semirigid rods, which are inserted into the corpora cavernosa. With this type of implant, the penis is always semi-rigid and needs to be lifted or adjusted into the erect position to have sex. It's less expensive and simpler than the inflatable, but the downside is that the man always has an erection, making certain social situations uncomfortable. The inflatable implant consists of paired cylinders, surgically inserted inside the penis and expanded using pressurized fluid. Tubes connect the fluid reservoir to a pump, which are also surgically implanted.

To gain an erection, the man presses on the pump, which has been implanted in the scrotum. The pump transfers saline solution from the reservoir to the cylinders in the shaft of the penis, inflating them and causing an erection. Pressing on a deflation valve at the base of the pump returns the fluid to the reservoir. Most men rate the pump as the best option in a bad situation. Still, having to squeeze your scrotum to literally inflate an erection is an awkward procedure within the context of sexual intimacy.

Again, this is not a *small* side effect of prostate cancer. But, like the incontinence market, the ED market is substantial. Given that penile-prosthesis implantation is the last resort for men with severe ED, the amount of money this procedure generates is shocking. According to Camille Farhat, president of American Medical Systems (AMS), a wholly owned subsidiary of Endo Health Systems, more than $500 million worth of penile implants are sold each year in the United States and $1.7 billion worldwide.[51] It's important to note that this extraordinary dollar figure only represents the cost of the unit, not the cost of surgery, which runs about $20,000.

Endo sees tremendous growth potential in the US urological market, due largely to our aging population. Remember, prostate cancer is a disease of aging. As I explained in chapter 3, the data show that men aged 60 to 69 have a 65 percent chance of having prostate cancer simply because of their age. The great majority of these men will die of something else other than prostate cancer; however, they make up a target-rich age group for the urology community. Another demographic that makes drug and device manufacturers in the prostate cancer industry happy is the explosion of baby boomers, people born between 1946 and 1964. The first wave of boomers turned 65 years old in 2011, which means they have arrived at the golden age that makes them permanent members of the "Medicare Club." The numbers are staggering. Medicare, which is on a glide path to insolvency, will have to handle an increased demand of 77 million boomers.

Speaking at an AMS mega investor day meeting in October 2012, Farhat noted, "Growing demand for its urological therapies are supported by the 'baby boomer' population explosion, providing us with a long run rate for growth." Farhat's slide presentation made clear that AMS is well positioned to dominate large sectors of the erectile restoration market, thanks to prostate cancer and the baby boomers.[52]

The radical-prostatectomy-driven ED market is irresistible for the drug and device industries. They have a ready-built market: tens of millions of Medicare-aged men, most of whom, as noted, have prostate cancer simply because they are 65 years or older. In essence, the prostate cancer industry is herding countless numbers of men via PSA screening into a system that renders them incontinent and impotent, creating new unnecessary clinical issues that produce more layers of profit. It is a great business model and the people in key leadership roles will continue to devise new strategies, not only to maintain their market, but also to expand it globally.

The AMS investor day presentation made no bones about the future of their urology sector, citing three key growth drivers: the erectile restoration business, accelerated growth in artificial urinary sphincter business in international markets, and expansion into "adjacent urology spaces," which simply means that AMS wants to exploit other areas on top of it incontinence and impotence products.

The cost to our health care system, especially the overburdened Medicare program, is catastrophic. Direct-to-consumer advertising is stitched into the fabric of the prostate cancer industry. Troll the Internet using search terms to find articles about incontinence or ED and hyperlinks will jump off the page, redirecting your attention to ads for brands such as Depend diapers or Viagra. Invariably, all these male-targeted ads feature a happy couple, always ready to play tennis or make love. And the ads always anticipate a happy ending for the men they portray.

More important is the human cost. Imagine the psychological and physical stress on a man who gets an "abnormal" PSA-test score, proceeds through the biopsy to radical prostatectomy, and is left incontinent and unable to have sex with his partner. As a last resort, he has a penile implant, which is not a surefire remedy to his problem.

Let me be clear: many men who have lost the physical ability to get an erection have benefited from penile restoration techniques, which are continually getting better. But there are inherent risks with any surgery, especially when foreign devices are surgically implanted in the body. If you go to the FDA's MAUDE site, there are more than 6,000 reported medical errors associated with penile implants, many of which are device failures. Below is a verbatim MAUDE report.

> EVENT DESCRIPTION:
>
> The device was removed due to a "device failure." As reported, the pump/cylinder set and connector from the assembly kit component only were removed and replaced with another pump/cylinder set. The reservoir component from the original implant surgery was left in place. 1/27/09 upon receipt of the physician/surgeon's operative report, he stated, "postoperative diagnosis: failure of penile implant with pain and curvature". Operation performed: explanation of company 3-piece implant with corporal body dilation and measurements and replacement of pump/cylinder set. Re-operative note: patient had a penile implant performed in 2010, which has become troublesome with pain and curvature. He has not been able to use the device due to pain. *He is thought to have problems with his cylinder which may be too large for his corporal bodies.*"[53]

I emphasized the last line of the MAUDE AE report to highlight the nature of the incident. This was a surgical error and it truly gives one pause. The surgeon implanted a cylinder that was too large for the man's penis, so that when he inflated it he had pain and curvature. Look at your pinky finger, and then imagine having a tube the size of your middle finger swelling inside your pinky. That's essentially what this man was going through, in a much more delicate body part. Reading through dozens of MAUDE reports, it is clear that most of the medical errors are device failures, leaks and ruptures being the most common. Infections and faulty placement of the devices also occur, but less frequently.

A SLIPPERY AND SHADY BACK ROAD

As examples of ancillary businesses sprouting from the prostate cancer business, I've briefly looked at artificial sphincters for incontinence and penile implants for ED. Both procedures are last resort-attempts at fixing the damage from a radical prostatectomy and, as I've stated, they have markedly increased the quality of life for many men. However, as I say throughout this book, it is the continuous supply of devices and physician marketing and direct-to-consumer marketing that is creating consumer demand. And, most of these products have little direct clinical worth. As pressure to curtail routine PSA screening grows, the prostate cancer industry is devising new-generation PSA tests that are "more accurate" (so it claims) in detecting prostate cancer, leading to fewer false positives. Since PSA is not prostate cancer-specific, this is no more than medical smoke and mirrors to keep the industry pumping new PSA tests into the market.

There are approximately 1,000 US companies in the high-tech medical industry, generating more than $64 billion in yearly revenue. The fields with the highest-grossing markets are spinal devices, cardiovascular devices, neuromodulator devices, diabetes devices, urology devices, and surgical technologies. An example of the device industry's rapid-fire production of new devices is the current concern voiced in a 2012 paper, "Primer: The Medical Device Industry." According to the author, Han Zhong, a growing regulatory burden is slowing the industry's projected growth. The growth-killer Zhong cites: "The average total time for the FDA to reach an approval through the 510(k) procedure has risen from 90 days in 2005 to 140 days in 2010, an increase of over 55 percent."[54] Think of that shocking statement. The device industry will suffer, Zhong says, because the FDA takes slightly more than four months to evaluate and approve a medical device.

There are currently several iterations of the PSA test awaiting FDA approval, which I'll discuss in an upcoming chapter. But one of the more aggressive additions to the line of tests is a new point-of-care PSA test called TrueDX, developed by True Diagnostics, Inc. Here's a snippet from its press release:

With the TrueDX™ PSA Test, doctors can immediately determine the PSA level in a patient with only a finger prick of blood rather than wait days for lab results from an intravenous blood draw. This unique test enables doctors to gain access to diagnoses in minutes and immediately create an effective treatment plan. The Company has a CE mark for a qualitative PSA test, TrueCX™ PSA, as a quick screen for over-the-counter use to determine PSA levels greater than 5.0 ng/mL.[55]

According to the media release, the company has received its CE mark, which documents a product's compliance for the clinical use of this type of technology. More telling is the point-of-care finger-stick blood test that eliminates the need for an intravenous blood draw and the time involved sending the sample to a laboratory. It seems that True Diagnostics is confident of FDA approval and is looking to simultaneously launch in the United States and Europe, possibly setting their sights on the massive Asian market as well.

Another new PSA test called the Opko 4KScore is already being used in the United Kingdom. Next stop, the United States. The test was developed and marketed by the US pharmaceutical company, Opko Health. It's being billed as a test that will reduce unnecessary biopsies by at least 50 percent. A headline in the British tabloid *Daily Mail* says it all: "SHOULD YOU HAVE THE NEW TEST FOR PROSTATE CANCER? FLAWS IN THE USUAL TEST LEAD TO NEEDLESS OPS THAT CAN WRECK SEX LIVES."[56]

Sex sells. Along with the mind-altering fear of the C-word, it is a mass marketer's dream.

Below the tabloid's headline is a picture of a man perched on the edge of the bed, head in hand, distraught looking. Behind him, his unfulfilled wife or lover stares vacantly at the back of his head, a picture of dejection. Her creamy skin and tow-colored hair blend her into the background of unrumpled sheets so that it makes her seem like she's fading away. It's typical British tabloid fare but it drives the message home: ED is a relationship destroyer and the 4KScore test will give you much better odds of avoiding the unnecessary situation this poor chap is in.

I asked Malcolm Mason, MD, an internationally regarded radiation oncologist at Cardiff University in the United Kingdom, about the second-generation PSA tests that are flooding the market. "There have been a series of important publications on reporting biomarkers and prognostic factors called PROGRESS guidelines, and all these 'fixes' would not pass that standard," said Mason, adding, "It's clear that there is a market for this sort of thing, and that must say something about satisfaction with the PSA test—if it was really good enough we wouldn't need all these other things."[57]

Peter Scardino, MD, a well-known urologist from Memorial Sloan-Kettering Cancer Center in New York City, gave this well-reasoned thought on PSA screening, during which he plugged the new 4KScore. That's not surprising, given the fact that Scardino is one of the developers of the 4KScore test and he's also a paid consultant for Opko Health.

> A diagnosis of prostate cancer requires a biopsy, and men should not have a biopsy without a good reason. PSA levels vary considerably and should be confirmed with a repeat test in six to 12 weeks before a doctor recommends a biopsy. In the future, new blood markers now in development such as free-to-total PSA ratios, the 4KScore and the Prostate Health Index (PHI) may be able to increase the accuracy of PSA testing in predicting the presence of cancer, especially aggressive disease.[58]

In a later interview, Scardino's loyalty to his test came through. "I believe this panel of tests [Opko 4KScore] will eventually replace PSA measures alone for the early detection of prostate cancer that needs to be treated, helping us to avoid dealing with small, indolent cancers that should be left alone."[59] Scardino's prediction that the 4KScore test will eventually replace the "old school" PSA assay should bolster Opko's stock prices. The financial investment blogger John H. Ford is super bullish about Opko's 4KScore, predicting that the test could generate close to $2 billion in annual revenue.

"Opko's CEO, Big Pharma guru Dr. Phillip Frost, has been *buying* large numbers of shares for the past couple of years. Given his remarkable track record, if he is buying shares in his own company, I pay attention," said Ford.[60]

The Pharma guru that Ford gushed over, Phillip Frost, MD, is a dermatologist whose meteoric rise in the pharmaceutical industry culminated while he was serving as chairman and CEO of Ivax Corporation. Frost sold Ivax to the Israeli-based Teva Pharmaceuticals in 2005 for $7.6 billion. According to *Forbes*, Frost also has stakes in close to a dozen firms, including the medical-device company SafeStitch, and Musclepharm, a company that sells athletes' apparel and supplements.[61] Leading up to the presidential election of 2012, Frost hosted a $50,000-a-plate dinner for Republican presidential candidate Mitt Romney in his Miami Beach mansion.[62]

Is it unscrupulous for a dermatologist to become a billionaire mover and shaker in the pharmaceutical industry? Of course not. We live in a free-market capitalist society that encourages entrepreneurship in the hope that it will incentivize the best and brightest among us to produce products and services that enhance society. But the inherent flaws in the system also entice a wide variety of players in health care to enter the drug and device industries and become fabulously wealthy by putting profit over the best interests of American health care consumers.

This charge is borne out not only by the PSA saga I'm writing about, but also by the manifest synergistic relationships between doctors and industry that have resulted in multiple scandals ranging from subtle advertising deception to blatant fraud. These unholy alliances go unchecked by the government oversight process, which in effect has become a de facto arm of the pharmaceutical industry.

I asked nationally regarded health care attorney and professor Christopher T. Robertson about Big Pharma's influence on the medical device industry. Robertson, who has researched and written extensively, said, "It is estimated that between 30 and 45 percent of the growth in medical spending is driven by the adoption of new medical technologies. This industry spends billions of dollars to create these products, but also spends about as much to change the behavior of prescribers, consumers, and payers to ensure they're purchased."[63]

I am convinced that the era of mass PSA screening is coming to an end, not only because of the inherent flaws in the initial FDA approval, but also because of the greed of the medical device industry (remember the four cruxes I spoke about in chapter 3, which explain the utter failure of clinical trials of PSA screening to date). That is, the industry will come up with new prostate cancer-detection tests that will simply supplant the PSA assay—with the same calamitous results. The vicious "develop and market the test without solid evidence" cycle is alive and well in American health care. We are seduced by elegant medical technology backed by clinical trials that are, for lack of a better word, rigged in favor of the drug and device industries. It remains an astounding and disturbing fact.

Pharma's slippery and shady back road to FDA approval is well documented, making efforts at better routes to approval all the more frustrating. Ben Goldacre, MD, author of *Bad Pharma: How Drug Companies Mislead Doctors and Harm Patients* hammered this point on page after page:

> The best evidence shows that half of all the clinical trials ever conducted and completed on the treatments in use today have never been published in academic journals. Trials with positive or flattering results, unsurprisingly, are about twice as likely to be published—and this is true for both academic research and industry studies."[64]

He goes on to say:

> If I toss a coin, but hide the result every time it comes up tails, it looks as if I always throw heads. You wouldn't tolerate that if we were choosing who should go first in a game of pocket billiards, but in medicine, it's accepted as the norm. In the worst case, we can be misled into believing that ineffective treatments are worth using; more commonly we are misled about the relative merits of competing treatments, exposing patients to inferior ones."[65]

For example, on Opko's website, you'll find a hodgepodge of cleverly crafted propaganda about the company's various products. There are links to clinical trials led by doctors with a vested interest in the products.[66] As I pointed out above, Scardino, for one, has become a public cheerleader for the 4KScore test. Frost and others make the incredulous claim that there are more than 750,000 unnecessary prostate biopsies performed each year on American men and that their product, the 4KScore, will cut that number by 50 percent. Adopt 4KScore and we'll save 350,000 men from needle biopsy, they're saying.

Like the standard PSA test, the 4KScore measures the total amount of PSA but also looks at three specific components of that number: "free" PSA, "intact" PSA, and human glandular Kallikrein 2, which is an enzyme that helps liquefy semen. The company explains that the test, using a "complex" formula, analyzes the relationship between the four biomarkers and gives a more accurate prediction of the need for a biopsy. Out with the old PSA test, in with the new.

While that sounds great, you have to ask: Where's the solid evidence for the medical claim that Opko's 4KScore test will prevent 350,000 unnecessary biopsies? An Opko press release cites evidence that is based on two old clinical trials that takes a lot of *creative* science to link with Opko's test.[67] Surely much more is needed; it has not been conclusively shown that the new test will have a positive effect on men's health.

But, as you've seen with the PSA test, a lack of evidence never stops anybody. Don't forget, Scardino (and his Sloan-Kettering colleague Andrew Vickers, PhD), invented the 4KScore test and is a paid consultant for Opko. Though disclosed, how can this not be a conflict of interest?

Of the thousands of medical-device companies in the United States, here are a few that are pumping various next-gen PSA tests into the marketplace: Opko Health, GenomeDX, Biosciences, Bostwick Laboratories, Metamark Genetics, Danaher, Hologic, Mitomics, Beckman Coulter, Genomic Health, MDxHealth, Myriad

Genetics, and Metabolon, and on and on and on. Is it any wonder that the device-industry representatives fret that the FDA has the temerity to take four months to approve a medical test, slowing down their conga line of prostate cancer-detection tests into America's $3 trillion health care pot of gold?

None of the aforementioned diagnostic tests have convincing scientific evidence supporting their clinical claims. Make no mistake about motive. This is all about money and the device makers are saturating the prostate cancer market with tests that have little, if any clinical relevance—certainly not enough to justify the $3,000 price tag on many of the newer tests. One irony attached to the next-gen group of prostate cancer-detection tests is that many of the former cheerleaders for the old PSA test are now jumping on the new-test bandwagon. The language is much the same as in 1986 and so are the results. None of these tests detect prostate cancer or accurately separate out the "turtles" (slow-growing cancers) from the "rabbits" (dangerous, likely-to-spread cancers).

Moreover, the rapid proliferation and approval of new tests indicates that the FDA has not learned a lesson from its mishandling of the Hybritech PSA assay. Dr. William J. Catalona summed up the prostate cancer-detection business environment with an amusing metaphor: "This field [next-generation PSA tests] is kind of moving like cell phones."[68] There is, of course, a major flaw in Catalona's analogy: unlike the whirlwind of new prostate cancer detection tests, cell phones actually do what they're purported to do.

As I noted in this book's introduction, confronting the embedded medical authority and the perverse incentives entrenched in our fee-for-service system is where the battle over the trust and value of American health care might very well be won or lost.

I HAVE AN INNATE MISTRUST of grand prescriptions for health care problems, but plugging some of the holes in the FDA approval process is a start—it would save money and lives. So would a heightened degree of healthy skepticism by American health care consumers. After all, we've been lied to before and the lies are usually powered by the synergistic relationships of industry, medicine, and marketing. While the misuse of PSA is the heart of this book, the theme of science for sale is generalizable across our system. You'd think that in this enlightened era of self-empowerment and digital connection that we'd be less vulnerable to the unrelenting promotional hype from industry that gave rise to the PSA health care tragedy. The fact is that we are not and the agencies that are charged with protecting American health care consumers are in tacit collusion with industry. It is science for sale on epic proportions.

Unfortunately, history repeats itself.

A glaring example is the Big Tobacco science-for-sale scandal. In 1956 Drs. Richard Doll and Bradford Hill published a study that demonstrated that smoking increased the risk of lung cancer.[69] Almost 50 percent of Americans smoked cigarettes at that time; however, public health organizations paid little attention to the study's culture-bucking findings. This was the era of *Mad Men:* everyone smoked—at work, in airplanes, and after sex. In response, Big Tobacco took the gloves off and geared up a rebuttal campaign, separating out groups for targeted advertisements—women, African Americans, working men. But the spearhead of Big Tobacco's pushback against the causal relationship between cigarette smoking and lung cancer was a veritable blitzkrieg using an ad titled "A Frank Statement," which touted the industry's scientific credibility.

Here's an excerpt from "A Frank Statement" as it appeared in the *New York Times* on January 4, 1954:

Recent reports on experiments with mice have given wide publicity to a theory that cigarette smoking is in some way linked with lung cancer in human beings. Although conducted by doctors of professional standing, these experiments are not regarded as conclusive in the field of cancer research. Distinguished authorities point out: There is no proof that cigarette smoking is one of the causes of lung cancer. . . . We believe the products we make are not injurious to health. To dispel concerns, we are establishing a joint industry group consisting initially of the undersigned. This group will be known as the TOBACCO INDUSTRY RESEARCH COMMITTEE. In charge of the research activities of the Committee will be a scientist of unimpeachable integrity and national repute.[70]

An excerpt from a highly regarded study titled "The Perils of Ignoring History: Big Tobacco Played Dirty and Millions Died" has chilling parallels to the PSA story.

The tobacco industry had a playbook . . . paying scientists who delivered research that instilled doubt, criticizing the 'junk' science that found harms associated with smoking, making self-regulatory pledges, lobbying with massive resources to stifle government action. A half-century of tobacco industry deception has had tragic consequences: Since the 'Frank Statement,' approximately 16 million Americans have died from smoking, and millions more have suffered.[71]

Sound familiar?

WHERE'S THE OUTRAGE?

In 1998 former US Surgeon General C. Everett Koop delivered a speech at the National Press Club titled, "The Tobacco Scandal: Where's the Outrage?" He said,

We have also learned that the tobacco industry recently paid scientists thousands of dollars to write letters to the editors of prominent publications to question the link between environmental tobacco smoke and lung cancer and to undermine the 1993 Environmental Protection Agency findings. This included one former NIH [National Institutes of Health] cancer researcher who was paid $20,000 over seven months to write to the lay and professional press. And when questioned he replied: "Are you getting paid for what you're writing? We're all out there working." Where is the outrage?[72]

I've been asking the same question for about three decades. Millions of American men who entered the PSA-test-to-radical-prostatectomy assembly line have had unnecessary, life-changing treatments: Where is the outrage?

The Big Tobacco science-for-sale scandal is perhaps, heretofore, the most notorious example of how an industry wields its deep pockets and political connections to promote its product. We've seen the story come full circle with the last cigarette commercial broadcast on January 1, 1971 at 11:59. It was a Virginia Slims commercial, and the slogan "You've come a long way, baby" is an example of just how deep into the consumer psyche industry goes to sell its products. Joe Camel and the Marlboro Man were shipped overseas, helping to capture the massive Asian cigarette market. Class-action suits followed, which put a public face to the victims of the tobacco industry. Remarkably, about 20 percent of American adults still smoke cigarettes. And lung cancer stubbornly remains the number one cancer killer for both men and women in the United States. To counter lagging sales in the United States, Big Tobacco uses its mega-money clout and promotion skills to exploit international markets. It is a human tragedy of epic proportions.

There's little worth in comparing tragedies. However, the decades-long misuse of the PSA test is worse in certain ways than the tobacco scandal. When I make that statement, it usually raises eyebrows being that tobacco is one of the deadliest carcinogens known to man. Inhaling cigarette smoke is poison and over several decades it will diminish your quality of life and likely kill you. But since at least 1966, Americans have been warned, right on the package, about the dangers of cigarette smoking. Every pack of cigarettes has one of many cautions, all shouting the message that cigarette smoking causes lung cancer. Despite the known harms of mass PSA screening—as evidenced by the strident warnings of the 1985 and 1993 FDA panels—nobody warned men about being manipulated into having a test that could lead to significant physical and emotional damage. In a following chapter, I'll begin putting human faces on the damage wreaked by population PSA testing.

So far, this chapter has dealt with distinct parts of the prostate cancer money chain. The scope of this book precludes extensive analytical examination of costs related to value. However, what I demonstrate is an identifiable corrosive element in the body of the multibillion-dollar prostate cancer industry: a parasite called greed. Proton-beam centers, with their $200 million price tag, and da Vinci robots, which cost $2 million, use prostate cancer as an important part of their business model without having persuasive evidence that the massive costs of these technologies milking our system are any better than less costly therapies. From the PSA test itself, all the way down the chain to Kimberly-Clark diapers for men and penile reconstruction, the prostate cancer business is a self-perpetuating industry that creates a need for services and products.

The PSA-screening debate has grown louder in recent years, but fixating on the PSA test obscures the greater issue and allows dozens more exotic new-generation prostate-detection tools to continue the same pattern of unnecessary treatments with the same results: millions of permanently damaged men. If we revisit the 1993 FDA Immunology Devices Panel meeting and go to the comment section after Catalona's presentation for Hybritech's PSA assay, panel member Dr. Harold Markowitz said, "I'm afraid of this. This basically, if it is approved, comes out with the imprimatur of the Committee. This goes out before the American public, and I think, as pointed out, you can't wash your hands of the guilt." Markowitz also mocked the idea of recommending that the PSA test came along with a package insert of instructions for primary care doctors, in effect, a tool to initiate a doctor-patient discussion about PSA. "How many physicians in practice read them? I suspect very few. It will basically be useless," said Markowitz.

The purpose of proposing an insert was to prevent wholesale mass screening. As Markowitz pointed out, it was a limp suggestion by panel members frantic to maintain their professional integrity. They wanted an escape clause, something that would wash their hands of guilt. But if actually used, what effect would an insert packet have? Let's see:

Before checking the PSA box on the blood-work panel, the primary care doctor says to his male patient:

> PSA does not detect prostate cancer, just abnormalities that could also be caused by a number of factors, sex for instance. An arbitrarily determined PSA reading might lead to a needle biopsy, which is generally safe, but can result in severe infection requiring hospitalization. The biopsy is not 100 percent accurate. But a positive biopsy might lead to a radical prostatectomy, which will leave you incontinent and impotent for an undetermined period. Oh, and there is also no evidence that having a prostatectomy will extend your life. So, should I check the PSA box?

First off, a primary care doctor does not have time for a conversation that requires a certain level of scientific understanding on the patient's part. Plus, laying out that gray area information would provoke a slew of anxiety-driven questions from a middle-aged man who only has one question: "Doctor, will the PSA test tell if I have prostate cancer?"

For the prostate cancer industry, ignorance is bliss . . .

MARKETING MEDICINE WALKS A FINE LINE

The word *quack* is derived from the archaic Dutch word *quacksalver,* which literally means "hawker of salve." In the Middle Ages quacksalvers hawked their faux cures in the market shouting in a loud voice. Medical quackery is the promotion of unproven or fraudulent practices. The Internet is the new market for quacks, hawking their salves.

But what is a quack? Defining quackery as promoting unproven therapies puts us in a bind. Pursuing ideas that break ranks with mainstream medicine has produced some of history's greatest medical breakthroughs. The preceding pages of this book surely illustrate that there is a level of uncertainty with all medical treatments. There is also a distinction between those who knowingly promote therapies that have no value and those who do so out of ignorance—or, in the case of PSA screening, those who are simply good soldiers following their marching orders.

Quackery in its purest definition is the multibillion dollar alternative medicine industry, largely promoted on the Internet and largely using cancer patients as the prime market. The sales pitch is great. Traditional medical practices—surgery, radiation, and chemotherapy—they say, do not cure metastatic cancer; there's no hope. And, to a large extent, that's true. On the other hand, what's documented about alternative medicine's track record in curing metastatic cancer is equally disappointing. One of the most famous cases of someone turning from traditional to alternative therapy was front-page news some 30 years ago. Tough-guy leading man Steve McQueen, the King of Cool, was suffering from mesothelioma, a rare form of cancer. He traveled to Rosarita Beach, Mexico, for a series of controversial treatments known as the Kelley Regimen. Named after its inventor, the orthodontist William D. Kelley, the most noted component of the treatment was laetrile, made from apricot pits. Kelley claimed to have cured himself of pancreatic cancer. After the treatment, McQueen publicly announced he was cured. The American Cancer Society worried that McQueen's popularity would send droves of cancer patients to the dark side of alternative medicine. But McQueen's resurrection was short lived; he died shortly after his announcement. However, prior to his death he made it known that the reason he sought out alternative therapy was simple: his traditional medical oncologist told him there was no hope for a cure.

The Kelley Regimen lies on the outskirts of alternative cures, but Steve McQueen's trip to Mexico for the regimen highlights the desperation of cancer patients who are facing death. Cancer offers a ripe market for exploitation. However, as I've discussed in previous pages, many mainstream therapies for prostate cancer offer hope without sufficient evidence to back up their claims. This is not quackery in the literal sense because cancer doctors are using therapies that have been approved by mainstream medicine, unlike so-called quacks that hawk cures that have not been vetted by rigorous

scientific method. Quacks aside, advocates of "alternative therapies" such as macrobiotic diets, herbs, and bioelectronics occupy the
higher tier of non-mainstream cancer treatments. Although positive
data for alternative medicine is scant to nonexistent, advocates point
to the dismal failure of mainstream chemotherapies in cancer. It's the
classic battle of two negatives, who wins?

Stepping away from the debate over alternative therapies and
mainstream treatments, the issue that speaks to the central theme of
my book is the profit-over-patient ethos that gave rise to PSA screening health disaster. And the bloated health care system itself is a
large part of the problem. Back in 1990, the US Government Accounting Office (GAO) designated Medicare as a high-risk program
because its size and complexity make it vulnerable to fraud, waste,
and abuse.[73] Further, since cancer is a disease of aging, the Medicare
program is a target-rich environment for back-office billing depart-
ments. According to the GAO, in 2009 the Centers for Medicare
& Medicaid Services (CMS), the agency that administers Medicare,
estimated billions of dollars in improper payments in the Medicare
program.[74] In the end, however, cancer patients are the pawns in
Medicare fraud and the other money-driven shenanigans that our
system encourages. People struggling against cancer are in an altered
state of mind as they move through life seeking a cure or some extra
time here on earth. The least they should expect is honesty from the
medical community, not a chess game of avoidance as their doctors
overbill Medicare for therapies that have insufficient proven benefit.

Frank Critz, MD, is the founder and medical director of the Radiotherapy Clinics of Georgia (RCOG), touting himself as "a leading
authority on prostate cancer treatment." According to his organization's website, Critz's "groundbreaking research has contributed
to the advancement of cancer research worldwide."[75] That's a bold
declaration. One thing is for certain, Dr. Critz is a world-class promoter of his clinics, which have made a lot of money treating prostate cancer.

One of Critz's claims to fame is a therapy he has been offering since 1979, which he has trademarked as "ProstRcision®." The

RCOG website claims that patients who undergo this therapy, in contrast to surgery, are far more likely to keep their sexual function and urinary control. A chart on the RCOG website sets out the "cure rate" of the clinics. One entry in the chart asserts that the ten-year cure rate in men with early, intermediate, and advanced prostate cancer who undergo "ProstRcision®" treatment is 83 percent. Blending the three categories together is confusing at best; it could lead men with advanced cancer to misunderstand their prospects. National statistics show that only about one-third of men with advanced prostate cancer live for five years.[76]

Critz and company have also made unusual statements such as, "While most doctors only talk about treating prostate cancer, Radiotherapy Clinics of Georgia physicians *specialize in curing it*."[77] The emphasized construction sounds like a used car pitch. But are doctors who are more cautious in their statements about what treatment can and cannot do to be avoided? I think not.

From the website, one could infer that ProstRcision is a unique technique for curing prostate cancer. In fact, the treatment involves the use of radioactive seed implants (called brachytherapy) and follow-up with external beam radiation to "make sure we get rid of the cancer completely."[78] Is this assertion backed by clinical results? As I've mentioned, PSA is naturally present in the healthy, benign, and cancerous prostate tissue. If you surgically remove the prostate you should have no PSA. The million-dollar question men ask after their procedure is: Did the treatment work? For men who have a radical prostatectomy, the definition of success is having a PSA reading of 0.1 ng/mL or lower. Ideally you want a zero reading. The million-dollar question, however, does not have such a clear-cut answer if a man has radiation therapy. There is no such PSA line in the sand that defines success. Unlike surgery, the effects of radiation therapy are gradual, sometimes taking up to three years for the PSA to hit rock bottom. Determining whether a man is cured of prostate cancer is a complicated and nuanced process. Critz's website states that they use the gold standard 0.2 ng/mL PSA level to determine cure. But in radiation therapy, there is no gold standard.

A trademarked treatment may sound impressive to a prostate cancer patient seeking his best chance for cure. But, according to nationally recognized urologist Gerald Chodak,[79] there's nothing unique about "ProstRcision®." "This is not a novel approach," Dr. Chodak has said. "In fact, many centers around the country offer the same treatment as long as they believe it's clinically appropriate [for the particular patient]. The problem is that it is so heavily marketed, the patient needs to be wary of misinformation."

Chodak continued, "For example, the center claims in its advertising that it has the highest proven cure rate for prostate cancer. That is simply not a fact based on good, well-controlled trials. To make comparisons of one radiation therapy over another is simply not possible in this day and age." Chodak stressed that the Agency for Healthcare Research and Quality has done a full analysis of all the well-done studies of radiation therapy. The Agency concluded that there is no proof that radiation therapy has better results or extends life more than active surveillance, and there is absolutely no proof that one form of radiation is better than another. "Attempts to claim the highest cure rates in the world is simply misinformation," said Chodak.[80]

This kind of problematic advertising is enabled by a toothless and overwhelmed regulatory system and a medical establishment that is addicted to tests and procedures. The fact that there are more than 240,000 newly diagnosed cases of prostate cancer each year in the United States; for most, treatment beyond active surveillance is unnecessary. But a culture of greed has grown up in the urology community. The prostate gland has become their golden egg. I've talked at length about tests and treatments that don't do what they purport to do. I've also pointed out how the culture of greed in the urology community drains our health care system of precious resource. Advertising pays dividends. Critz and his colleagues have never had a shortage of patients, many of whom are Medicare recipients.

However, on April 3, 2012, the Department of Justice Office of Public Affairs released a public statement that RCOG and certain affiliates paid $3.8 million to settle a false claims case, with no admission of any wrongdoing. According to the Justice Department, Critz's clinics allegedly "billed Medicare for medical treatments for prostate cancer patients in excess of those permitted by Medicare rules and for services that were not medically necessary." The complaints were filed separately by two whistleblowers. The Justice Department added, "it was alleged that the practice overbilled Medicare for physician consults (production of complete special consultative reports for an individual patient) and for pre-plans ordered by Dr. Critz that were not medically necessary and/or never reviewed by the doctor."[81] The RCOG group made the settlement payments and moved on. Critz's clinics are still up and running.

There are about 240,000 new patients in the United States every year, and urologists compete aggressively for their share of those men. Within my lifetime, I've seen a consistent shift to the type of commercialism that you have just read about. Although Gordon Gecko in *Wall Street* says "Greed is good," it is an addiction, and there never seems to be enough money to satisfy its appetite.

In medicine, we are at our best when dedicated to solving the dazzling array of scientific puzzles that demand cures and life-changing advances. Our great difficulty is to moderate our urgency when it comes to cancer with well-reasoned patience. It is worth repeating stories of failure in which a rush to approval led to poor results that cost lives and money. Lessons need to be learned. Sometimes it is important to become a detached spectator, and put emotion on the sidelines.

FROM P$A TO DEATH

The expression "a drowning man will grab the edge of a sword" is an appropriate way to introduce the story I'm about to tell. Like most professors, I read myriad journal articles, many of which are written simply to accommodate the "publish-or-perish" ethos that is part of life as an academic. Every so often, I come across a piece that stands out. In 2012 an article in the *Journal of the National Cancer Institute* (*JNCI*) did just that. Telling about it will underscore points

I've made about the ineffectual approval process that floods the market with drugs and devices that do more harm than good. Also, in a way, it's a micro-narrative of my 30-plus year struggle advocating against the use of routine PSA screening.

I've spoken at length about legions of men irreparably harmed by unnecessary treatments for prostate cancer. I've used the "turtle and rabbit" analogy to explain the clinical dilemma in prostate cancer— we still cannot identify an indolent cancer from one that kills. It is a merciless ambiguity that we struggle to find answers for.

Each year, about 30,000 American men will die of prostate cancer. It is an especially cruel death—the main site of metastases in prostate cancer is bone, which causes severe pain, fractures, spinal cord compression, and a rapid degradation of quality of life. Seeing a once-vital man shriveled into a fetal ball, looking up with that hollow-eyed thousand-yard stare of despair, sticks in your heart. As you'll see, dying men at the far end of the prostate cancer spectrum also offer a rich market for industry. It's a group of men drowning in cancer who will grab the end of a sword.

Prostate cancer is classified as an adenocarcinoma, or glandular cancer. It begins when normal prostatic fluid-secreting prostate gland cells mutate into cancer cells. During the early stages of cancer, tumors are typically benign, remaining within the margins of a tissue. As the tumor grows and becomes malignant it gains the ability to break down cellular boundaries and invade other tissue, a process called metastasis—literally meaning "new place." A lining called the capsule covers the prostate gland and once the cancer has moved beyond the capsule, the prognosis is grim. There is presently no cure for advanced prostate cancer; oncologists try to extend the patient's life for as long as possible.

A clue for extending the lives of men with prostate cancer was discovered in the late 1920s by a Scottish physiologist named Charles Huggins. He was interested in glandular secretions and the secretion of his choice was prostatic fluid. At the time, it was known that estrogen controlled the growth of female breasts. Huggins hypothesized that male hormones controlled the growth of the normal prostate gland. Following his scientific nose, he experimented on dogs, noting that when he removed their testicles, prostate tumors began to shrink. This line of inquiry is long and complex, but it proved that prostate cancer was hormone-dependent. Therefore, obstructing testosterone production should halt the growth of a prostate tumor.[82]

Early-stage prostate cancer is treated with local therapies. One standard treatment is testosterone-lowering drugs. As Huggins' dog research proved, deprive the prostate of testosterone and the cancer becomes dormant. It works, but only temporarily. And despite minutely low testosterone levels, the cancer progresses and the terminal phase of the disease stakes its claim on the body. These men become what are known as castration-resistant and their survival is about two to three years. There are only a few options left for such patients and they all have significant side effects. These men and their advocacy groups are desperate for a miracle drug or at least something that offers extended life without the brutal side effects of chemotherapy.

In 2007 researchers thought they found such a treatment and, as with PSA, a tidal wave of false hope spread throughout the prostate cancer community. This story is long and convoluted, so I'll tell the part that most pertains to this book. The paper I read in *JNCI* was titled "Interdisciplinary Critique of Sipuleucel-T as Immunotherapy in Castration-Resistant Prostate Cancer." Admittedly, it is not a very eye-grabbing title. But after I read the abstract, a sense of déjà vu took hold. The paper's lead author, a trained scientist named Marie Huber was contending that an FDA-approved indication did not do what it purported to do. Huber has argued that the data actually suggest that the Sipuleucel-T (Provenge) treatment "is harmful for older men and, at best, does nothing for men under 65."[83] Although the decades-long PSA disaster is magnitudes greater in terms of the physical and financial damage, the fundamental profit-over-patient theme is similar.

This story began with hope for late-stage prostate cancer patients in the name of a therapy called Provenge, developed and marketed by the biotech company Dendreon. I'm sure you've seen it advertised on

TV. A healthy-looking middle-aged man grabs a wrench and tackles a leak under the sink as his adoring wife looks on, smiling. Then the voiceover: "People can count on me to get the job done. So when my prostate cancer returned, my doctor told me that this time it can be different, with Provenge, a personalized treatment that lets me count on my own body to fight back."[84] The commercial tugs at your heart-strings. It portrays a man who is still vital, who still has relevance in the world. He loves his wife and he has a grandson that he wants to see graduate at least from high school. These are elements of being human that everyone can attach to. But Huber's *JNCI* paper and her extensive follow-up research and publications, tell a very different story about Provenge.

You'll recall that as an immunotherapy, Provenge is designed to stimulate the body's immune system to be more effective at destroying cancer cells. Provenge was developed for men whose prostate cancer stopped responding to the medications that suppress testosterone. As mentioned, in clinical terms, these men are castration resistant—they have entered a darkened room in their long battle with prostate cancer.

In the 1970s, groundbreaking research showed that the immune system could attack cancer cells by using many of the same techniques it uses to fight infection. Scientists sought to harness that power. In theory, it's better than injecting the bloodstream with poisonous chemotherapy drugs. For one, it's less toxic, so patients can tolerate a longer treatment cycle. Simply put, our immune system is a network of cells, tissues, and organs that have evolved to defend our bodies against invading pathogens. For example, pus is a protein-rich whitish-yellow fluid that consists of a buildup of spent leukocytes (white blood cells) from the body's immune system in response to infection. That's your immune system at work.

All cells carry a set of surface proteins, identifying markers. Most prostate cancer cells have high levels of the protein prostatic acid phosphatase (PAP). Remember that PAP was mentioned at the 1986 FDA advisory meeting. Dendreon had asserted that the PAP protein is specific to prostate tissue, so it would try to "train" the immune system to attack prostate cancer cells bearing PAP. Theoretically, it would slow the growth of the cancer and prolong survival. However, as elegant as the theory is, delivering Provenge therapy is a complicated and costly process—$93,000 per patient annually.

Provenge is "manufactured" individually from each patient's cells. First, blood is drawn from a vein and passed through a machine that separates the desired white blood cells, or leukocytes. This process of harvesting specific cells is called leukapherisis. The rest of the blood and cells are returned to the patient. Then, the collected leukocytes are shipped to the Provenge manufacturing facilities where they are purified to remove any stray cells. The purified cells are mixed with an activating substance called an antigen and incubated at 37 degrees Celsius for about 48 hours.

After incubation, the cells are washed and shipped back to the doctor's office to be re-infused into the patient. This process is done three times over two weeks to complete the treatment. Remember, the process involves transporting bags of human cells that need to be infused into patients the day they arrive, so scheduling and timing has to be exact, which can be very stressful for the doctor and the patient. All men receiving Provenge have terminal prostate cancer, so it's worth the stress and inconvenience, as long as the treatment does what it's purported to do. As you continue reading, try to put yourself in a desperate patient's head.

The Provenge story has three basic components: money, politics, and the clinical part. It is a complicated tale filled with Wall Street shenanigans and FDA cover-ups. To avoid losing the core issues, I'll boil the story down to its basic constituents, beginning with Mitchell H. Gold, MD. After graduating from Rush University Medical School in Chicago, Gold did a urology residency. But it doesn't appear that he practiced very long before entering the pharmaceutical industry. With his perpetual tan and a salesman's grip-and-grin hard-charging attitude, Gold worked his way into leadership roles in several companies. In 2001 he signed on as Dendreon's president and CEO. His name would soon be wedded to Provenge's tumultuous and controversial road to FDA approval.

Provenge was being hyped as a miracle treatment for men with terminal castration-resistant prostate cancer. Emotions were boiling even before Dendreon applied to the FDA for a biologics license, a request for permission to market a drug. Advocacy groups had circled their wagons, demanding that Provenge be approved. According to groups like Care To Live, men were dying by the thousands as FDA dragged its bureaucratic feet. (Some of the members of Care to Live were Dendreon investors. They were among the promoters of the drug who created a climate of fear, warning of dire consequences if Provenge was not approved.) The drug-approval procedure is similar to the process that Hybritech's PSA test went through: clinical trial data are presented to persuade an FDA advisory panel—in this case the Office of Cellular, Tissue, and Gene Therapies Advisory Committee—to vote for approval. However, getting FDA approval for incredibly expensive cancer drugs is far tougher than for medical devices. As in medical devices, the FDA is not bound by its advisory panel's recommendation to approve or disapprove, but the agency generally follows the panel's lead. For drugs like Provenge, which cost hundreds of millions of dollars to develop, the critical FDA advisory meeting is where they live or die.

At the time Dendreon was seeking approval for Provenge, the story was one of the hottest topics in Wall Street watering holes. Huge money is wagered on cancer drugs. Traders on the Street were holding their collective breath, waiting to see whether Provenge got the thumbs up from the FDA. Dendreon CEO Gold was upbeat about the chances for approval, citing a very positive pre-meeting discussion with the FDA. Wall Street runs on money and emotion. One off-the-cuff remark from someone in the know can send a stock on a roller-coaster ride. In 2005 Jim Cramer, the wacky over-the-top host of CNBC's *Mad Money* disparaged Provenge's chances for approval with his usual corny sound effects and histrionics.[85] The stock became a candle in the wind. Public apologies followed. The drama was in full stride as the long-awaited FDA meeting got underway on March 29, 2007.

In many ways, it was reminiscent of the 1993 FDA panel meeting for the PSA test. The room was packed with advocates, injecting pure emotion into a scientific meeting with huge consequences. This is a quote from Carl J. Rosapepe—an advocate from the US Too survivor support group who spoke last—as he pleaded for approval: "It is not the nature of science to be perfect. No studies are perfect. None yield 100 percent results. It is the nature of science to be sound, to give us excellent probabilities with honest representation and to serve humanity. Today you bring us the science. We bring you humanity. We ask that you approve Provenge. Thank you."[86]

Thunderous applause!

The FDA Office of Cellular, Tissue, and Gene Therapies Advisory Committee voted 17 to 0, endorsing Provenge as reasonably safe; it voted 13 to 4, endorsing the trial data as showing substantial evidence the drug is effective.[87] Dendreon, stock investors, and prostate cancer patient advocacy groups celebrated, believing that FDA approval was right around the corner. After the panel recommendation, Dendreon's stock rocketed from around $5 per share to $23.58. In a move that raised eyebrows in the investment community, Gold sold a big chunk of his holdings, cashing in for several million dollars.[88]

Why would Gold sell stock in a company that he had nurtured into maturity, right when its stock value seemed destined for a veritable moon shot? Maybe he had a crystal ball. Another investor also cashed in at the same time as Gold. Businessman Steve Fleischman, who was a prostate cancer patient, activist, and stockholder in Dendreon, sold an undisclosed amount of his holdings. Fleischman was reluctant to talk about his windfall, but in a moment of frank introspection he said, "The sad thing is that Dendreon became more of a stock play than a humanistic play—a game between long and shorts—and all about padding people's pockets."[89]

Then the other shoe dropped.

On May 9, 2007, about five weeks after the FDA meeting that seemed so favorable to Provenge, Dendreon received a complete response letter from the FDA demanding more conclusive clinical trial data before its drug could be approved. In a very rare case, the FDA went against its own advisory panel that had overwhelmingly voted for approval, abruptly putting Provenge on hold for several years while Dendreon accumulated more convincing data. The advocacy community went nuclear, decrying the FDA's decision as a death sentence for thousands of desperate men. A miniseries of drama unfolded. There were threats of violence and charges of conflicts of interest involving two advisory panel members who had voted against approval—Howard Scher of Memorial Sloan-Kettering and Maha Hussain of the University of Michigan. Were there, in fact, conflicts of interest? Or was this a conspiracy theory hatched by overwrought prostate cancer advocates? The answer is: both.

Like most influential and well-connected academic oncologists, Scher and Hussain had strong ties with select pharmaceutical companies. For instance, Scher was the lead investigator for clinical trials financed by the drug companies Novacea and Schering-Plough on treatments that were in direct competition with Provenge. While one cannot reduce the complex relationships in the cancer-drug-development world into a conflicts-of-interest editorial, it is impossible to separate high-powered cancer doctors like Scher from the pharmaceutical industry. Here's a partial list of Scher's relationships in Pharma: he's a paid consultant for Veridex, Aragon, BMS, Exelixis, Foundation Medicine, Genentech, Medivation, Amgen, OrthoBiotech Oncology Research and Development, Dendreon, Enzon, Millenium, Novartis, Roche, and Sanofi-Aventis. He also owns stock in several biotech companies and receives research funding from a half dozen others.

In the FDA disclosure form it came out that Hussain's husband had considerable stock holdings in drug companies whose drugs competed with Provenge. Frankly, it would be difficult to find many nationally regarded oncologists who didn't have some financial relationship with Big Pharma. Being a paid drug company consultant is business as usual in the hierarchy of oncology, making conflicts of interest somewhat ubiquitous.

The situation was further inflamed when Scher and Hussain articulated their opposition to Provenge in scathing letters to the head of FDA's oncology drug division, Richard Pazdur, MD,[90] an imperious, rail-thin man who to this day is much maligned by the advocacy community as an impediment to life-saving cancer drugs. We'll never know if Scher's opposition to Provenge was in some way influenced by his dealings with competing drug companies. What we do know is that the letters he sent to Pazdur clearly articulated legitimate concerns about the effectiveness of Provenge and how the favorable results were obtained.

When the letters were leaked to the press,[91] they fueled outrage that culminated in a lawsuit by the advocacy group Care to Live. It alleged that Pazdur, the FDA oncology drug czar, intentionally placed Scher and Hussain on the advisory panel in an attempt to rig the votes against Provenge because he knew they stood to benefit significantly from a decision not to approve the vaccine.

It went from bad to worse.

There were more threats and nasty blog posts. The Securities and Exchange Commission's (SEC) Office of the Inspector General looked into charges that insiders had manipulated Dendreon's stock. In a grand swipe, advocates accused the FDA of torpedoing Provenge so that a new era of immunotherapies would not threaten the multibillion dollar chemotherapy industry. Full-page ads were taken out in national newspapers. Prostate cancer advocates from Care To Live organized a raucous demonstration at FDA headquarters.[92] As in most situations driven by raw emotion, any legitimate beefs were lost in the mayhem of name-calling and ridiculous accusations. Characters like junk-bond-king-turned-felon-turned-prostate cancer-survivor-advocate Michael Milken joined the fray.

The Provenge story, once so full of hope, had turned into a train wreck.

Let's flash forward a few years to April 29, 2010. After reviewing new Dendreon data, the FDA finally announced that it had approved Provenge for men with advanced prostate cancer. Remember that in 2007 Dendreon's CEO Mitchell Gold sold a chunk of his holdings right before the initial FDA decision to reject Provenge. Three years later, Gold sold more than $28 million of Dendreon stock. In a filing with the SEC it was disclosed that, just hours after the FDA announced it had approved Provenge, Gold exercised options on 270,625 shares that had been purchased at a price ranging from $4.41 to $9.77 per share. He sold them for $51.01 per share. The following day, Gold sold another block of stock, for a cool $28,878,927.[93]

Timing, as they say, is everything.

Other Dendreon insiders made millions on April 29, 2010, too. Stockholder Fleischman was right when he said that "Dendreon became more of a stock play than a humanistic play."[94] For some, at least, it was indeed all about padding their pockets.

Provenge was supposed to be a story about offering hope to desperately ill men facing imminent death. Instead, Gold and his cronies turned it into a story of greed and arrogance. There were so many characters and subplots involved it would read like a tawdry Russian novel.

Now to Marie Huber.

For several years Huber was a general analyst for a registered investment firm. In her spare time, she began learning about developments in health care, with a particular interest in new treatments coming out of the emerging field of immunology and cancer. Her endgame was to find interesting investment opportunities in biotech and medical-device companies for her firm's clients. Huber was aware of the Provenge saga; the controversy surrounding its path to FDA approval seemed too tendentious to be deemed an appropriate investment for the firm's conservative clients. But the promise of a new therapy that harnessed the immune system and didn't have the harsh side effects of chemotherapy intrigued her.

Provenge had gained approval largely on the strength of its phase III study called IMPACT (Immunotherapy for Prostate Adeno Carcinoma Treatment). To Huber's dismay, there was very little publicly available evidence to support the positive results proposed by Dendreon. The IMPACT trial consisted of 512 patients with advanced prostate cancer. They were split into two groups: one group received Provenge, the other group, called the control arm, received a placebo.[95] The men getting Provenge lived about 4.1 months longer than the men receiving a placebo, which might not seem like something to cheer about, but in the cancer world, four months is considered a significant benefit.

However, the closer Huber looked, the murkier the picture became. For one, the complicated history of changing endpoints and enrollment criteria had left the evidence Dendreon presented to the FDA with severe flaws. Endpoints are what clinical trials use as their way to measure a drug's success or failure. Some examples of endpoints are survival, improvements in quality of life, relief of symptoms, or disappearance of the tumor. In Dendreon's pre-IMPACT trial of 127 men, the investigators used the endpoint time-to-progression—that is, after the cancer is treated, how long it takes for the tumor to start growing again. It works this way. At the beginning of the trial, the patient's prostate cancer is measured by scanning tests. As with the IMPACT clinical trial, in this first study the 127 men were spilt into two groups—Provenge and placebo. They were monitored to see which group's tumors progressed at the slowest rate. It's a tricky endpoint and as you've read, the FDA declined to approve Provenge in 2007, when the first trial failed to show that it slowed tumor growth.

This is important. In round two, Dendreon changed its endpoint for the IMPACT study from time-to-progression to overall survival—the percentage of people in a study who are still alive for a certain period of time after starting treatment. The study was designed so that a statistically acceptable survival comparison of the two groups could be done after at least 304 men died.

At a JPMorgan health care conference in San Francisco, Dendreon CEO Gold announced that 304 men on the IMPACT trial had died. Using a football analogy, Gold said, "This is a very exciting time for us and for patients. We're on the 10-yard line, we're in the red zone and we've got to punch it into the end zone now."[96]

Sports metaphors have their place, certainly in the blood sport of American politics, but not in medicine, not after you've reached your goal of 304 dead men.

The final results from the IMPACT trial were published in the *New England Journal of Medicine (NEJM)* on July 29, 2010, three months after Provenge was approved. Dan Longo, MD, a former cancer immunologist at the National Institutes of Health who is now deputy editor of the *NEJM,* wrote an editorial that appeared in the same issue. In comparing men in the Provenge group and the placebo group, he said it was "hard to understand" how the men taking Provenge could have lived longer "without some apparent measurable change in the tumor, either evidence of tumor shrinkage or at least disease stabilization reflected in a delay in tumor progression." This lack of "tumor effect," Longo went on to say, "raises concerns that the results could have been influenced" by something else, what he characterized as "an unmeasured prognostic variable that was accidentally imbalanced in study-group assignments."[97] However, it is worth noting that while the objective of conventional cancer therapy, e.g., chemotherapy, is to shrink the tumor, vaccines work differently and take longer to show their effect.

In any event, Longo questioned whether Provenge was responsible for making the men live longer, because the drug had no measurable effect on the cancer. So what was, in fact, going on? What was influencing the results? This is what Huber wanted to know. In fact, the question had also been raised by Scher in his famously leaked 2007 letter to Pazdur in which he gave a host of reasons why Provenge should not be approved. In closing, Scher wrote, "All of the difficulties cited, and the investigator's own conclusions, show how there are simply *too many alternative explanations* for the observed survival difference" [emphasis added].[98]

The advocacy community pilloried Scher for opposing FDA approval. He was characterized as a scientific collaborator, a player of sorts who fell in league with Big Pharma. Mudslinging aside, Scher's concern about alternative explanations had validity, as Huber would come to believe.

Typically, within two to six months after the FDA approves a new therapy, it posts on its website large sets of internal documents related to the trial. When posted, Huber began examining them. That's when the red flag went up. Huber unearthed what she believed was an alternative explanation for why the men receiving Provenge lived four months longer than the men receiving placebo. She pursued her alternative explanation, culminating in the *JNCI* article I mentioned at the beginning of this section.

Undeterred by critics, Huber proposed an alternative explanation from thousands of pages of documents, many of which were heavily redacted. As you recall, the underpinning of Provenge therapy is a process called leukapheresis, in which the patient's blood is drawn and put through a machine that harvests a special type of white blood cells. The cells are then transported to a Dendreon manufacturing plant where they are incubated with a specially marked antigen that helps the immune system target and kill cancer cells. The processed cells are then transported to the doctor's office and re-infused in the patient. Provenge was approved because the IMPACT trial showed that the men receiving Provenge lived 4.1 months longer than the placebo group. They did, but Huber's analysis comes up with an eerie conclusion: The men on the placebo arm died sooner, because the placebo itself killed them. How? Huber contends that during the re-infusion process the placebo group received 20 billion fewer white blood cells than the men on Provenge. Plus, many of the white blood cells they did receive were—because of faulty handling—dead or dying.

It is an unthinkable, yet plausible theory.

Huber has stated publicly that if you return dead and dying cells to men you are likely to cause inflammation, which can stoke the growth of cancerous cells.

The most logical explanation of the data I've seen is that Provenge treatment is harmful for older men and, at best, does nothing for men under the age of 65. In the production of Provenge, more than 90 percent of a man's circulating white blood cells are harvested, 65%

are lost in manufacture, and 35 percent are returned. Patients lose 20 billion cells whose normal role is to suppress their cancer.[99]

Dendreon insists that Huber's data are flawed and that Provenge has helped thousands of men with prostate cancer. Huber has been attacked on all fronts for her alternative explanation. Moreover, her pleas to the FDA have been rebuffed. Both the FDA and Philip Kantoff, MD, the lead author of the IMPACT trial, have derided Huber's investigation as post-hoc statistical analyses that "are exploratory and must be interpreted with caution."[100] And why is post-hoc analysis irrelevant? With other drugs and devices, there's been a history of mistakes and scientific fraud that's been exposed after initial publication.

Not only has the FDA stonewalled Huber, but doctors treating prostate cancer patients with Provenge have clammed up as well, "refusing to go on the record about the treatments and doctors making $7,000 per prescription won't even engage in a discussion about whether the vaccines helps patients," said Huber.[101]

Huber has never stated that her alternative explanation is an absolute truth. To my knowledge, she has no ax to grind to color her objectivity. A telling comment about Huber's alternative explanation came from one of Dendreon's paid consultants, nationally regarded statistician Donald Berry, PhD, of M. D. Anderson Cancer Center: "The control [group's placebo] vaccine used in IMPACT and in the predecessor trial had never been used anywhere for anything and may well have been detrimental to patients. Here's a great way to get your drug approved: Kill the control patients."[102]

Despite huge challenges, Dendreon forges ahead. Europe is a still an untapped market. The following snippet from an internal Dendreon message board pretty much describes the corporate philosophy about targeting urologists:

Dendreon is seeking a Urology Key Account Manager who will be responsible for maintaining and developing long-term client relationships in large, influential Urology practices. . . . They will continually develop their skills ensuring that they produce a sales volume at or above the assigned key account sales quota. This position will also raise the profile of Dendreon in the relevant urology community and influence sales growth in urology markets within a territory.[103]

All Huber wants is an honest scientific inquiry to prove or disprove her claim. If she is right, it means that some prostate cancer patients are being harmed by the very treatment they believe is helping them. It also means that the color of money obscured the true mission: developing treatments for men with prostate cancer who have run out of options. According to Huber, dismissing her theory was one of many attempts to smokescreen the truth while Dendreon insiders made millions even though Provenge has never lived up to the company's financial expectations, but not for a lack of trying.

When it's all about money, things go wrong. On August 4, 2011, Dendreon's second-quarter results fell far short of Wall Street expectations, sending the company's stock over the cliff. At the close of the market, the stock had lost nearly 68 percent of its value. The company's investors lost millions and they felt betrayed. On March 13, 2013, Dendreon signed off on a $40 million securities class-action lawsuit filed by investors who alleged that the company misled them about its finances, business operations, and prospects for Provenge.[104] Making matters darker were the plaintiffs' allegations that company insiders collectively sold nearly $86 million of stock before it crashed, including about $35 million by one co-defendant, former chairman and CEO Mitchell H. Gold.

I'll be clear, I'm not promoting Huber's theory that the placebo shortened the lives of the older patients on the IMPACT study, thus creating an artificial 4.1-month longer survival for the men receiving Provenge. But I do believe that this is something that needs to be looked at by a process untainted by special interests. During the writing of this book, it became public knowledge that Marie Huber was engaged in an ethical and SEC legal issue, which has since been settled. These matters are separate and apart from this discussion on Provenge, and should not detract from its scientific and therapeutic importance. Her theory remains alive until it is disproved. Given Provenge's controversial road to FDA approval and Dendreon's history of insider Wall Street deals that ended in a messy class-action suit, I think it's fair to conclude that money, not the survival of desperate prostate cancer patients, was the company's underlying endpoint. Once again, the FDA's failure to lead played a major role in this very sad story.

In the roiling debate over health care, it would be hard not to exaggerate the staggering failures that have been produced by unchecked power and greed. Most men who rise to the top of medicine and industry have a touch of the Icarus complex, Type-A personalities who don't recognize any limitations. Our system enables them to run free in their desire to achieve success and material goods. It becomes an idealized goal that blinds them to the harm their ambitions leave behind.

Another thing that would be hard not to exaggerate is the power of emotion to sway sound scientific judgment. As was the case with the FDA's approval of the PSA test for screening, which is the start of all that has followed, prostate cancer advocacy groups rallied and lobbied tirelessly for Provenge's approval. They branded anyone who questioned the evidence as a traitor to men with prostate cancer. In the Provenge story, emotion and money won. What about the patients?

FIVE

U̶N̶INTENDED
CONSEQUENCES

*We have it. The smoking gun. The evidence. The potential weapon
of mass destruction we have been looking for as our pretext of
invading Iraq. There's just one problem—it's in North Korea.*

—Jon Stewart

I want you to stonewall it.

—Richard Nixon, Presidential Transcript,
March 22, 1973

The American Civil War was the bloodiest conflict in our history.
The chaos and killing and political rancor were also marked by
massive fraud, particularly within the meaty target of Union
war contracts. Most agree that the fraudulent sale of sick mules to
the Union army was, in part, the catalyst for the federal False Claims
Act, also known as the Informer's Law or the Lincoln Law.

The False Claims Act empowers private citizens with knowledge
of fraud against the government to file a whistle-blower or qui tam
action on behalf of the government. Naturally, there's financial, personal, and professional risk involved. So to encourage whistle-blowers,
the False Claims Act originally awarded 50 percent of the amount

recovered to the relator (the person who brings the action and provides the facts on which it is based). Today the relator's share is less, approximately 30 percent, and the action must recover at least $1 million.

The lone maverick who blows the whistle on a greedy entity bilking the government and harming innocent citizens has been the dramatic model for scores of books and movies. For instance, the risk of whistle-blowing was documented in the Academy Award-nominated film *Silkwood,* based on the life of activist Karen Silkwood, who raised concerns about corporate practices related to the safety and health of workers in a nuclear facility. Silkwood, armed with documents, was on her way to meet a reporter for the *New York Times* when she was killed in a mysterious car accident. The documents, which were the smoking gun, were missing from her car. Another award-winning film, *The Insider,* starring Russell Crowe, was based on a true story aired in a *60 Minutes* segment about Big Tobacco whistle-blower Jeffrey Wigand. In a nutshell, internal documents leaked from Big Tobacco revealed that the companies knew that the chemical properties of nicotine made it highly addictive, in direct contrast to their executives' testimony before Congress in 1994. To prove that the CEOs from Big Tobacco perjured themselves, Wigand and the government set up a qui tam action that opened the floodgates for class-action lawsuits.

The central component to any False Claims Act action is called the smoking gun—the object or fact serving as evidence that fraud or a crime was committed. The phrase traces its roots to a Sherlock Holmes story, "The *Gloria Scott,*" in which Arthur Conan Doyle described a murder scene: "We rushed into the captain's cabin . . . there he lay with his brains smeared over the chart of the Atlantic . . . while the Chaplain stood with a smoking pistol in his hand."

The original *60 Minutes* story on the Big Tobacco cover-up was aired in 1995. However, much to the distress of the whistle-blower, Jeffrey Wigand, who had stuck his neck out, the televised version was highly edited at the orders of CBS owner, Laurence Tisch, who controlled the Lorillard Tobacco Company.[1] Although the unedited story was eventually aired a year later, Tisch's sanitizing of the original piece illustrates how even a heralded investigative program like *60 Minutes* is not immune from the influence of power and money.

NO SMOKING GUN

In 1983 my former associate at the Millard Fillmore Hospital in Buffalo, Dr. Maurice Gonder, asked if I'd like to join him at the State University of New York at Stony Brook on Long Island, New York, where he was chair of the Urology Department. At that time I was at Cook County Hospital in Chicago, doing mostly service work and the position at Stony Brook offered me a chance to get back to pure scientific research. So I accepted, pulled up stakes, and moved east.

During my house hunt, I was referred to the law firm of Glynn & Mercep to represent me in the purchase of my new home. We entered into an agreement and over time both partners became familiar with my work and my discovery of PSA. In 1997 Tim Glynn went to see his primary care doctor for a checkup. There was no glaring symptom he could put his finger on, he was simply in a bit of a funk. A PSA test was part of the routine workup and during his physical exam Glynn was told that his PSA was slightly elevated. "My doctor referred me to a urologist who recommended a biopsy. I asked him if I could wait and have another PSA test, just to make sure, but he said I should just get it done to be safe."[2]

Glynn consented to the biopsy and, after two anxious weeks of waiting, his urologist informed him that he had prostate cancer. The doctor recommended a radical prostatectomy, as soon as possible. Glynn remembered the mind-numbing period that followed, a universal sensation men share upon hearing the C-word—a sense that your world was spinning out of orbit. "The urologist was candid," Glynn recalled. "He said it's a four-hour operation and I would lose three pints of blood." The doctor was equally candid about the post-op side effects of incontinence and impotence, but he assured Glynn that they were treatable. "This guy was telling me that he's going to cut out my prostate gland, charge me 20 grand, and then treat the side effects, which are his bread and butter. I actually thought, wow, urology's a great business."

Instead of marching into the operating room, Glynn called me, seeking advice. After explaining the various issues concerning his diagnosis, I arranged for him to go to the Crittenton Hospital in Michigan to see Drs. Duke Bahn and Fred Lee, pioneers in the then new field of interventional radiology. This medical subspecialty of radiology uses minimally invasive image-guided procedures to diagnose and treat diseases. The first step in treating prostate cancer is determining whether the disease is confined to the prostate. Because tumors need a blood supply in order to grow, Lee and Bahn used color-flow Doppler imaging, which color codes various structures and functions in the prostate. Red indicates blood flow and helps pinpoint the location and extent of the tumor. They determined that Glynn's cancer was confined to the prostate, which allowed him his first sigh of relief since his initial diagnosis.

When Glynn returned with the good news, we had several more conversations about his treatment options. Although he was taking his time and processing the information, thinking about foregoing surgery, he had entered the cancer gulf, a place that too often has more questions than answers. Unanswered questions are open-ended luxuries that those with cancer cannot afford.

In deciding on next steps, there were a number of things for Glynn to consider: his wife, his career, and his law partner. As far as we've come in bringing cancer out of the closet, there is still a stigma attached to the disease. His partner was worried about him, not only for his long-term health but also how the cancer would affect his ability to work in the high-pressure field of law. Glynn tried to factor in lifestyle issues. He was only 48 years old at the time. He was an avid sailor, yachting in the Virgin Islands for five weeks a year. He also played a good game of tennis, enjoying the rush of competition. He rethought the urologist's discussion about side effects and wondered if having surgery would make physical passions a thing of the past.

But ultimately his wife's panicked urging to get it out prevailed and Glynn decided to have a radical prostatectomy. I put him in touch with H. Ballentine Carter, MD, at Johns Hopkins, who, to my knowledge having been mentored by Dr. Patrick Walsh, was one of the best prostate surgeons in the country. Glynn was a tall, vigorous man who radiated the confident presence of an athlete and I felt that Carter would give him the best chance of preserving his sexual function and the vitality that goes with it. Even though Carter characterized the surgery as successful, Glynn later confided that although he felt healthy, he was a changed man; a part of him he couldn't quite describe had faded away.

Over time he grew angry, feeling that his urologist had misled him about the actual clinical value of the PSA-testing process.

Recalling our conversations—particularly my explanation of why the PSA test does not do what it purports to do—Glynn decided that there was adequate justification for legal action against the companies that manufactured and marketed PSA tests for the early detection of prostate cancer. After consulting with his partner, Glynn began the laborious process of launching a qui tam or whistle-blower action, with me as the relator. We met at his office with other attorneys of the firm and began building a case. I had volumes of documents I'd collected over the years, offering proof in support of my own earlier studies and observations that the PSA test did not do what it had been approved for, as an aid in the detection of prostate cancer.

The basis of the action was that the federal government was being soaked for incredible sums of money in Medicare, Medicaid, and VA payments for unnecessary prostate biopsies and the consequential treatments, all of which were driven by mass PSA screening. Glynn's and my premise—based on my discovery of PSA in 1970 and follow-up studies—was that the PSA test did not do what it was marketed to do, namely detect prostate cancer. And the companies knew this all along; therefore they were defrauding the government.

After several meetings, Glynn filed the qui tam under seal and served a copy to the US attorney. I was the plaintiff-relator "to recover treble damages and civil penalties pursuant to the 'False Claims Act' on behalf of the United States of America against 16 pharmaceutical companies, collectively known as the defendants."[3] The claims in the action are "founded on the Defendants' false claims, false statements and fraudulent misrepresentations in promulgating, disseminating and manipulatively advertising various forms of assay kits for the detection of prostate-specific antigen."[4]

The qui tam action was a thoroughly researched document that laid out a damning case against the defendants. We proved that the PSA test kits were no better at predicting prostate cancer than biopsying a random sample of men over the age of 50 from a telephone book. (With one male turning 50 approximately every 10 seconds, the market for prostate screening is growing at an extraordinary rate.) The document Glynn and his associates prepared with my help was a searing indictment:

> The Defendants (monolithic pharmaceutical giants), displaying corporate ethics more commonly found in the tobacco industry, seized upon the perfect marketing strategy to sell their Assays: the most fearful word in the English language, CANCER. By dint of celebrity endorsements, hidden sponsorships, and an insidious advertising campaign . . . the Defendants have created a stampede for the use of their products, "a fervour which would not disgrace a medieval inquisition."[5]

"Filing a qui tam is 'a pig in a poke'; we knew that going in," Glynn told me. "But the government actually took an interest. I'm sure the damages we totaled in the action caught their eyes. Starting in 1994, when the test was approved for early detection, we estimated the United States suffered damages at $8 billion per year, or $80.0 billion trebled, which came to $240 billion. When we finished totting up all the unnecessary procedures, we're close to a trillion dollars in damages. We had a few preliminary meetings with attorneys from the US District Court for Eastern New York." On the strength of those meetings they sent the qui tam up the chain to the

Justice Department in Washington, DC. "The Feds were interested," said Glynn. "They, then, to move the ball forward, flew up an attorney from the Justice Department with who, together with two local representatives from the Justice Department, had a follow-up meeting during which we went through all of the allegations in the qui tam action, item by item."

They questioned me on every scientific allegation in the qui tam action. It was a grueling process during which I had to rigorously defend the science and Glynn had to justify how his legal arguments made a strong false claims case. Glynn explained, "Dr. Ablin truly convinced the Feds that these companies had wangled the science and defrauded the government, big time. They went back to DC leaving us feeling very good about the prospects of a major settlement. But then [a government attorney] met with one of my associates, Larry Kelly. Larry came back from that meeting looking shell-shocked. He said the Feds had dropped the action. Dumbfounded, I asked why, and he said, 'they told me on the "QT" that the fraud component of the action was unsupportable.'" Glynn explained that in legalese it's called "justifiable reliance," which simply means that one party is justified in taking action based on the statements of another party. However, the FDA knew that there was little evidence of effectiveness and significant evidence to the contrary, but for some reason they approved the PSA test anyway. As such, an essential element of fraud required to support a qui tam was missing.

Glynn summed up the disappointing outcome. "You won't find any internal notes on that conversation the Feds had with Larry. They aren't the sharpest knives in the drawer, but they're not stupid either. . . . Months of work down the tube. But the real kicker was that Big Pharma got away with a trillion-dollar fraud."

The men who were damaged got lost in a number with so many zeros. The Justice Department agreed that the science I presented was irrefutable. It was sitting on one of the biggest false claims actions in medical history and they were champing at the bit to ramp up the action. Then the bottom fell out. The FDA knew the whole time that the PSA test was, in effect, an elegant medical sham driven by greed and facilitated by a broken and corrupt regulatory system.

Ironically, the FDA itself ended up being the smoking gun.

BIG UROLOGY DOES A 180

Will the real American Urological Association (AUA) please stand up?

The AUA is one of the most powerful medical lobbying groups on Capitol Hill. Not surprisingly, Congress is a captive audience for prostate cancer advocacy. Men hold most of the seats in the House of Representatives and the Senate; their average ages are 57 and 62 years old, respectively, making them an irresistible environment for prostate cancer advocates angling for leverage and funding. But as with many policy issues ballyhooed on Capitol Hill, the AUA has flip-flopped on its PSA messaging, adding more confusion to an already dangerously tangled health care issue. Yet the group seems to want to walk away, guilt free, from a disaster it helped create. It's left a visible trail; let's follow it.

In 2000 the AUA's Expert Panel concluded that routine PSA testing should be offered to all men age 50 years and older. If a man had increased risk factors (family history, for example, or African American heritage), the AUA recommended that PSA should be offered to men between 40 and 50. If the PSA level was 4.0 ng/ml or more, the AUA said that a biopsy was "indicated."[6]

In 2009 the AUA lowered the PSA threshold. More men should have the test, they said, recommending that it be offered to "well-informed men aged 40 or older who have a life expectancy of at least 10 years. The future risk of prostate cancer is closely related to a man's PSA score; a baseline PSA level above the median [that magic but arbitrary 4.0 ng/mL] for age 40 is a strong predictor of prostate cancer." Note the inclusion of that phrase "well-informed men"; it's pointed, because most men are not even aware they are getting their PSA tested; it's just part of a routine physical, done without any discussion as to the implications.[7]

On May 3, 2013, the AUA updated guidelines on PSA screening once again.[8] But this time they sent shockwaves throughout the prostate cancer community. The latest guidelines recommended against PSA screening in men between the ages of 40 to 54. And for men aged 55 to 69 years old, the AUA recommended that the decision to undergo PSA screening involve a conversation about the potential harms associated with the test. The guideline also recommended not screening men over age 70. Guideline panel chair, H. Ballentine Carter, MD, offered this assessment of how we arrived at this point in the PSA debate. "The public is very enthusiastic about screening, partly because of our messaging. The idea that screening delivers benefits may have been over exaggerated."[9]

For years, the AUA had been the chest-thumping 800-pound gorilla in the room when anyone dared challenge the validity of PSA screening in the general population.

If implemented, the AUA's new recommendation would certainly have a chilling effect on the number of PSA tests given every year in the United States, which is currently about 30 million. Those 30 million tests lead to more than a million biopsies, which lead to upward of 100,000 prostatectomies that are not proven to increase a man's chances of survival but can devastate a man's quality of life. If we had a graph to depict the use of PSA testing and the incidence of unnecessary procedures from 1986 until today, the two lines would converge at its plot point—the AUA, the FDA, and the medical-device industry. In explaining its policy U-turn, the AUA stated that it employed a different analytic process to write its 2013 guidelines. Instead of consensus opinion, the AUA panel relied on a systematic review of evidence from the scientific literature, citing the same 2009 studies referenced by the US Preventive Services Task Force in 2012, when it issued its recommendation against PSA screening.

But here's the whiplash moment: before the ink on the 2012 task force recommendation had even dried, a furor of criticism was publicly hurled at it. Leading the charge: the AUA. The group shot out a press release, saying it was outraged and believes the Task Force is doing men a great disservice by disparaging what is now the only widely available test for prostate cancer . . . we hold true to our current position as supported by the AUA's "PSA Best Practice Statement" that, when interpreted appropriately, the PSA test provides important information about the diagnosis, pre-treatment staging, or risk assessment of prostate cancer patients.[10]

Remember, the task force is a nonpartisan group of physicians whose sole purpose is to analyze all the currently available scientific information and make recommendations on preventive services such as PSA screening. Citing an 80 percent rate of false-positive PSA tests, it concluded that there was a "moderate to high certainty the service has no net benefit or that the harms outweigh the benefits. A better test and better treatment options are needed. Until these are available, the [task force] has recommended against screening for prostate cancer."[11]

The AUA continued to fight back hard. It launched a letter-writing campaign, hitting all the big media outlets, from the *New York Times* to the *Wall Street Journal, USA Today,* and the mainstream TV morning shows. It was an aggressive, full-court press to counter the task force's recommendation. And it delivered its message as a direct gut punch: The task force recommendation against PSA screening, the AUA asserted, was tantamount to a death sentence for thousands of American men.[12]

How could the AUA fiercely condemn the 2012 task force's recommendation against routine PSA screening and then turn around one year later and essentially agree with it? Was it some kind of religious conversion? In 2009, when the AUA had recommended routine PSA screening for 40-year-old men, the exorbitant harms associated with population screening were already well documented.[13] In 2004 Thomas Stamey, MD, an early proponent of PSA screening released a highly anticipated study in the October issue of the *Journal of Urology* in which he concluded, "The PSA era is over in the United States. Our study raises a very serious question

of whether a man should even use the PSA test for prostate cancer
screening anymore."[14]

But back then, the AUA wasn't ready to give up its position.
As late as 2012, the AUA hosted the fourth annual "Know Your
Stats" National Prostate Cancer Awareness Campaign, partnering
with the National Football League (NFL). The campaign's website
boasts that over the past four years they "have reached more than
305 million men and their families, urging men to talk to their doctors about PSA screening."[15] The sponsor for the 2012 "Know Your
Stats" campaign was Intuitive Surgical, the company that developed
and markets the da Vinci Surgical System that has virtually taken
over the radical prostatectomy business. You can draw your own
conclusion about this relationship.

I asked Paul D. Abel, MD, a well-known British prostate specialist for his take on why, in 2013, the AUA adopted a new outlook
on PSA. "There wasn't any new evidence that would have impacted
the AUA's decision to change its PSA guidelines between 2012 and
2013," he told me, "so it seems that they were simply finding it increasingly difficult to justify their position."[16]

Asked what effect he thought the AUA's guideline shift would
have on PSA screening, Abel said, "It seems unlikely that the AUA
guideline changes will have any impact at all on medical practice, at
least at the present. Fewer or no radical prostatectomies means no
income, or retraining, for individual surgeons, at least in systems
like you have in the US, and that's a sobering thought!"[17]

In my view, the AUA was making a transparent effort to stay
in front of the PSA-screening disaster. It issued a guideline that attempts to please everyone but ends up mired in ambivalence. Most
striking was its raising of the age for initiating PSA testing from 50
to 54. Even for those who still believe in the value of PSA screening,
this makes no clinical sense. According to mortality data, 46 percent
of all men between the ages of 50 and 59 have prostate cancer, making the 50 to 54 age bracket a worthless charade of appeasement.
Once I unpacked their long and rambling document, it was clear that
the AUA was scrambling in the backfield to avoid being sacked. And

once again, American men and their primary care doctors were on the sidelines, scratching their heads over what to do next.

To me, the AUA's nuanced messaging of its updated PSA guidelines is nothing short of an admission of guilt. As Abel said, "they simply cannot justify their position,"[18] so the AUA offers a well-reasoned capitulation. In reality, it's a self-indulgent form of indifference and the men who were treated like medical poker chips are paying the price of that indifference, paid for in millions of damaged bodies.

Of course, the AUA is just one of the important Big Urology players in the PSA drama. In 1989, five years before the PSA test was approved as a cancer-screening tool, the pharmaceutical giant Schering-Plough found a backdoor way to supercharge the market for their PSA test. (Recall that, at this point, the FDA had only approved use of the PSA test to monitor men with prostate cancer, so any other use such as screening was considered off-label.) Schering-Plough paid the advertising firm Burson-Marsteller $1.2 million—a huge amount for the time—to launch Prostate Cancer Awareness Week. The goal was to aggressively promote PSA screening with a blitz of fear-mongering ads and free screening campaigns.

Prostate Cancer Awareness Week exploded, becoming the nation's largest screening program in history. From its inception, the number of screening centers increased from about 100 to more than 1,800 in 1992—an 18-fold increase in just three years! In 1996 more than 800 centers provided free PSA tests.[19] Burson-Marsteller managed Prostate Cancer Awareness Week's national media efforts until 1993, when the Public Relations Unit of the University of Colorado Health Sciences Center took over. It immediately enlisted retired General Norman Schwarzkopf as the bullhorn for PSA screening. Appearing on the cover of *Time* magazine and dozens of national TV shows, he grabbed the nation's attention and, with his inimitable swagger, "ordered" men to get their PSA test. Who's going to disobey Stormin' Norman?[20]

There was only one tiny fly in Schering-Plough's ointment: under the federal Food, Drug, and Cosmetic Act, it's illegal for a medical-device maker to promote off-label use of a product. At their discretion, a doctor can prescribe a medication, device, or test off-label, but companies that promote such use are breaking the law and face severe criminal and civil penalties. However, that didn't happen here. Although Schering-Plough was never punished for its PSA PR blitz, in August 2006 it agreed to pay $435 million in fines and plead guilty to criminal conspiracy charges filed by the US Justice Department for various infractions, including the illegal off-label promotion of a cancer drug. It was Schering-Plough's third multimillion-dollar settlement for illegal drug promotion in five years.[21] For Schering-Plough, paying a few-hundred-million-dollar fine is like fishing out spare change from underneath the sofa cushions. The company has also been accused of misconduct, such as bribing doctors to prescribe their drugs and infiltrating large medical practices with their own company-paid doctors.[22] The company is a repeat offender thriving in a revolving-door regulatory system.

Illegal, arrogant, cynical. That sums up the mindset of Big Pharma. It's all about the prostate cancer market, not about the men.

The main players in the prostate industry long had every reason to know that routine PSA testing in healthy men has no clinical benefit and causes significant harms. In 1993, when Hybritech sought approval for its PSA test in early detection, Steven Woolf, MD, spoke on behalf of the US Preventive Services Task Force, saying,

> The Task Force has determined that PSA screening fails to meet the criteria for effective screening. The test lacks accuracy in detecting early stage disease. There is little evidence that early detection of prostate cancer improves patient outcomes and there is mounting evidence of the adverse effects of testing and treatment, which range from patient anxiety and discomfort to the substantial physical complications of surgery, such as incontinence, impotence, and even death. The FDA decision on the PSA test, by setting off a wave of national screening, would ripple through the health care system in the form of increased biopsies, prostatectomies and radiotherapy. This has broad financial implications for urologists, pathologists, radiologists, radiotherapists,

administrators of hospitals and clinical laboratories, pharmaceutical companies, the manufacturers of the PSA test and many other
interests. The lives of millions of American men will be negatively
affected.[23]

And, they were. Remarkably, the task force issued a similar
warning in 2012, more than 20 years after it first advised against
routine PSA screening. Given the scientific facts about the limitations of PSA, it is unconscionable that no action was taken to subdue
mass screening of perfectly healthy men.

But there's a simple explanation: fear of public retribution.

According to Michael L. LeFevre, MD, the vice chairman of the
task force that issued the report, in 2009 he and his fellow panel
members had voted to recommend against PSA testing, but knowing they would have to defend themselves against the inevitable
firestorm of criticism—from the AUA and advocacy groups—they
slowed the process down, issuing their recommendation three years
later in 2012.[24] Internal documents reveal that in 2009 the task force
was ready to issue a "D" rating, which recommends against PSA
screening in healthy men of any age, but the task force was still lick-
ing its wounds from an earlier attack for its recommendation against
routine mammograms for women aged 40 to 50 years—so it quietly
put PSA on the backburner.[25]

A year later, in November 2010, just before the midterm elec-
tions, then task force chairman Ned Calonge canceled a review
meeting, once again delaying a PSA recommendation. Politics may
have played a heavy role: Calonge and others felt that recommending against PSA screening might rub some pols the wrong way and
jeopardize future funding. Kenneth Lin, a central researcher on the
PSA review panel resigned in protest.[26]

How many men might have been spared an unnecessary life-
changing radical prostatectomy during that delay?

"I will take full blame and full credit," said LeFevre.[27] His ad-
mirable honesty aside, LeFevre's statement is startling. Think of it: a
dedicated doctor working for a government task force admitting that

he and his colleagues delayed a public health warning because they were afraid of blowback from the urology community and other stakeholders in the prostate cancer business.[28]

LeFevre's admission speaks to the culture of fear promulgated by the prostate cancer industry. And in this instance the industry won. Between 2009 and 2012, it obtained a three-year window of opportunity during which more than 3 million more men had painful needle biopsies and about 300,000 of those men needlessly had their prostate glands cut out of their bodies. Fear of the AUA and other powerful entities in industry and the advocacy community created this grim medical reality.

On at least one occasion, the AUA has also cashed in on the off-label marketing of PSA tests. I'll elaborate on that in the upcoming section because it adds more proof that the AUA's vested financial interest in population PSA screening has been the reason for the decades-long public war on anyone who challenged PSA.

This is a good place for me to move into the next section of this chapter. So far we have discovered that the FDA was fully aware that the PSA test it approved in 1994 had no clinical value in detecting prostate cancer; its accuracy was comparable to a coin toss. We also move to the next section with a clearer picture of AUA's financial relationship to the PSA-test franchise. Moreover, in chapter 6 we'll look at a very basic right of American health care consumers, and how it was deliberately flouted.

FAILURE TO WARN

In 1960 Ralph Nader read that automobile crashes were the fourth leading cause of death in the United States behind heart disease, cancer, and strokes. He was determined to find out why. His research led him to a singular conclusion: the law placed far too much emphasis on driver error and not enough on the lack of safety features in the automobile manufacturing process.

Over the decades, Nader became an iconic figure; his life's work has been dedicated to a simple premise: the government's primary role is protecting its citizens, not only from external forces such as terrorism, but also from the perils of our free-market system.

One of Nader's famous consumer advocacy cases focused on the undisclosed handling problems of a compact car, the Chevrolet Corvair. It culminated in the groundbreaking book, *Unsafe at Any Speed*. Nader insisted that consumers have a right to know if the products they purchase are reasonably safe and effective. When consumers are left in the dark about obvious product dangers, it constitutes a failure to warn in legal parlance.

To win a failure-to-warn case in a court of law, a plaintiff must prove that the missing warning was a substantial factor in the injury. In other words, if there had been adequate warning, the plaintiff would have altered his or her conduct. Establishing a relationship between the manufacturer's failure to warn and an injury means proving causation, which is a tough legal challenge. I have served as an expert witness in several malpractice suits, and the burden of proof is always a steep hill for the plaintiff to climb.

Is the FDA liable for a class-action failure-to-warn case in reference to the PSA test? In 1985 the agency ignored its own advisory panel, which was troubled by the potential for misuse of the PSA test. The advisers had sent a crystal-clear message: an approval of the Hybritech PSA test as a monitoring tool for men with prostate cancer must be strictly enforced. After a contentious closed-door session, Dr. Harold Markowitz, the panel chairman, warned: "A number of people have been unhappy with the product . . . a lot of the group, if not all, feel there should be very strict limitations in the wording of the product concerning predictive value."[29]

The advisory panel was acutely aware that Hybritech had a perhaps not-so-hidden agenda: get the go-ahead to market their test as a monitoring device of the thousands of men already in treatment for prostate cancer, and then mount an assault on the market they really wanted: the 30 to 40 million healthy men who could be screened annually for prostate cancer. This is where the big money was to be made. And indeed, a year or so after the 1986 approval of the test as a monitoring device, PSA screening of healthy men gathered steam. The FDA had to know about Schering-Plough's Prostate Cancer Awareness Week, which was, at least in part, a drive to promote off-label PSA use, yet the agency did nothing about it.

Where was the warning?

But let's give the FDA a pass on that early period of the tragedy and move up to 1994, when the agency finally approved the Hybritech PSA assay for early detection—the only PSA test in the country with that indication. At the time, FDA panel member Markowitz warned of dire consequences if the PSA test is approved and used as a mass screening tool on the American public. The consequences of unnecessary biopsies, surgeries, and life-altering side effects would spiral out of control.[30]

And, as Markowitz forewarned, with the imprimatur of the committee, medical-device companies began cashing in with such aggressive marketing that the FDA finally had to respond.

In 1995, seeking to address concerns about widespread off-label use of PSA assays other than the Hybritech Tandem PSA test, which was the only FDA-approved PSA test for use in the detection of prostate cancer, Bruce Burlington, director of the FDA's Center for Devices and Radiologic Health, sent warning letters to laboratories across the nation: "Clinicians ordering PSA tests should become familiar with both the intended uses and the diagnostic outcomes which would be expected using a particular assay," he wrote.[31] In the letter, Burlington said that the FDA is "aware that some clinical laboratories are using PSA tests, approved only for monitoring patients who have been diagnosed with prostate cancer, to screen for prostate cancer in undiagnosed patients." He stressed that the safety and effectiveness of this off-label use had not been established. Note the timid language. Burlington said the agency was aware that some laboratories were using PSA tests off-label. It takes more than some laboratories to process some 30 million PSA tests a year!

As pointed out in the July 17, 1995, issue of *The Gray Sheet*— a weekly newsletter that covers the medical-device and diagnostic industries—device manufacturers had little incentive to seek FDA approval of their PSA tests: the widespread and unchecked off-label use of the tests already existed. Hybritech estimated that about 90 percent of all PSA tests sold at that time by industry were used off label for early detection of prostate cancer.[32] What with the PSA test free for all, Hybritech was posting dismal sales numbers, down by more than 20 percent. Ironically, the competition was drowning the company that had first opened the PSA floodgates.

Incredibly, as it turned a blind eye to Schering-Plough's Prostate Cancer Awareness Week screening-for-dollars binge, the FDA stated that the agency had no reason to believe medical-device companies were actively promoting their PSA tests for off-label use. Instead, the agency placed the blame squarely on the shoulders of the medical community, which was certainly an easier target than Big Pharma. But, there was enough blame to go around and, as you'll soon see, industry and the medical community were equal partners in the unholy alliance of promoting off-label PSA screening for profit.

By the way, staffers at the FDA said that the warning letters sent to the medical laboratories were meant to increase awareness about the potential dangers of off-label use and that there would be no further action.[33] Burlington's letter also noted that along with the issue of off-label use, the many different PSA tests on the market "may produce different results on the same specimen depending on the antibodies and the reaction conditions used in each particular assay."[34]

So the FDA was actually saying that the accuracy of the PSA test you've just bet your manhood on is essentially arbitrary. If there is one overriding message that jumps off the pages of the FDA communications, it is a sense of total detachment. It writes warning letters, carefully crafted so as not to offend, and then moves on. As I read the letters, I never felt the agency had any sense of conviction, or that the officials in that bureaucracy truly understood the gravity of the situation in human terms.

Three years later, under mounting pressure the FDA sent out more warning letters about the extravagant off-label use of PSA tests. One of the more telling letters was written to Bayer Corporation, saying that it was in violation of section 201(h) of the federal Food, Drug, and Cosmetic Act, which prohibits a company from promoting off-label use of a medical device.[35] Bayer, like scores of other device makers, was selling its PSA tests to laboratories to be used in screening, although it was only approved "as an aid in the management [monitoring] of prostate cancer patients." It was also placing ads where its advertising buck would get the biggest PSA bang, in journals such as *CAP Today,* a publication of the College of American Pathologists. That makes sense. It also placed ads in the *AUA Daily News,* which is the newsletter of the AUA. To the point I made earlier about AUA's financial ties to the PSA-test franchise: on the surface, it wouldn't seem inappropriate for the AUA to generate revenue through paid advertisements; most media outlets derive a substantial income this way. But the AUA, America's largest and most respected urological association, was benefiting through these ads, in which Bayer illegally promoted the off-label use of the PSA test.

These ads triggered the FDA to take action, albeit limited. What follows is an excerpt from the warning letter sent to Bayer on August 25, 1998:

The ads that we reviewed appeared in the June 1998 issue of Clinical Laboratory News, in the May 31–June 4, 1998 issues of the AUA Daily News and in the April 1998 issue of CAP Today. The ads in Clinical Laboratory News and the AUA Daily News say, "Competitors offer free and total PSA assays. Wouldn't it be better to measure the cancer-specific component directly?" The other ad says, "The simple truth is that measuring only complexed PSA is truly simple" and "At Bayer Diagnostics, we are currently developing a more specific method than either total PSA or the free-to-total ratio."[36]

With regard to the first Bayer ad, the Office of Device Evaluation has advised us that *it is not accurate to claim that there is a cancer-specific component for prostate specific antigen (PSA). At best, PSA is organ-specific.* It is known and it has been demonstrated by the data that appear in Bayer's 510(k) for the device, that complexed PSA occurs at low concentrations in men with normal health. It is inaccurate, therefore, to claim that complexed PSA is cancer specific since it is present in normal men . . . *Implying that your device can be used to detect prostate cancer has, as described below, changed the intended use of the device. It has also, consequently, made an unfounded claim of superiority over the products legally marketed for those uses.*[37]

That snippet is frustrating on several levels, especially the italicized sentence. Since discovering PSA in 1970, I've publicly repeated those same words—PSA is not cancer-specific; therefore it has no value as an early detection tool in the manner used. The FDA knew this in 1994 when it approved Hybritech's PSA test for early detection. As cited during the qui tam action, the FDA had full knowledge that PSA has no value in detecting prostate cancer, not only from my initial observations[38] but ironically, as mentioned in chapter 3, from the very scientists associated with the development of the PSA test. Its studies in the early 1980s showed that PSA was not cancer specific,[39] making the test inappropriate for screening.

Here's FDA's stern warning for Bayer's illegal promotion of off-label PSA tests:

You should take prompt action to correct these violations. Failure to promptly correct these violations may result in regulatory action being initiated by FDA without further notice. These actions include, but are not limited to, seizure, injunction and/or civil penalties.[40]

What you have read up until now has presented damning evidence that several powerful entities have knowingly misused the PSA test to generate huge profits. For one, the pharmaceutical-device-making industry—as evidenced by Schering-Plough's back-door promotion of PSA screening—has illegally promoted mass PSA screening by its promotion of off-label tests. It was enabled in this by the weak-kneed response of the FDA. Using warning letters, or for that matter, million-dollar fines to dissuade profiteering by pharmaceutical powerhouses is akin to thwarting an elephant's charge with a BB gun.

More disturbing is the FDA's passive-aggressive participation in this national tragedy. Charged with ensuring that the nation's medical products are safe and effective, the agency approved a device that has caused incalculable harm and suffering for millions of healthy men. Then we have the AUA. The fact that this medical association would take money from a company promoting the illegal use of a PSA test speaks volumes about the connection between money and the reprehensible mass marketing of PSA.

Moreover, the FDA's utter failure to properly regulate the use of the PSA test created an environment perfect for exploitation, not unlike a city besieged by looters during a blackout. A 2001 survey found that about half of large life insurance companies required PSA testing of all male applicants aged 50 and older. Laboratories seized the opportunity. LabOne, a testing laboratory in Lenexa, Kansas, performed a whopping 60 percent of all US PSA testing for insurance companies. On its website, LabOne stated, "The majority of cancers detected by an elevated PSA are aggressive cancers. PSA does not detect latent, or slow-growing cancers." This assertion, as you know from previous discussions about PSA, is scientifically false. Even the company's vice president and chief medical director, Dr. J. Alexander Lowden, admits that the claim is false. "It [the statement] really shouldn't be there. [But] it's written for underwriters who are nonmedical people . . . and what we're trying to do is sell [PSA] tests."[41]

THE FEAR FACTOR

I've spoken about the type of fear conditioning marshaled by the prostate cancer industry to herd men into PSA screening programs. In chapter 6 you'll meet an eclectic group of men who were confronted with a prostate cancer diagnosis. Their reactions are a panoramic view of how the C-word affects decision making. First, however, I want to introduce two men whose experiences shed light on the outer edges of the PSA story. For one, fear was employed as a weapon to silence his free speech; for the other, fear changed the way he practiced medicine.

MICHAEL WILKES, MD, is a popular professor at the University of California, Davis (UCD). He is also a nationally regarded prostate cancer expert. He originated what's known as the innovative doctoring courses that are now used by 33 medical schools across the country.[42] Wilkes is a terrific doctor and teacher by everyone's assessment. On September 28, 2010, UCD sponsored a men's health seminar that prominently advertised "Prostate Defense Begins at 40." Also conspicuous was an advertisement for the AUA's collaboration with the NFL, the "Know Your Stats" campaign. The event highlighted the special guest, Guy McIntyre, a three-time Super Bowl participant. It was a testosterone-fueled event with one underlying purpose: to promote PSA screening.[43]

When Wilkes first learned of the event and promotional campaign on September 16, 2010, he e-mailed the proper authorities at the UCD Medical School, expressing concern about the presentation and the lack of objectivity by the AUA regarding PSA screening, which he characterized as "far away from evidence-based." Wilkes did not attend the men's health meeting, but two medical students recorded the event and gave him the tapes. One student commented that the meeting was "unabashed marketing" and that the urologists "mentioned that having a baseline PSA at age 40 predicted lifetime risk of prostate cancer."[44]

On September 30, 2010, Wilkes published a powerful op-ed piece in the *San Francisco Chronicle* titled "PSA Tests Can Cause More Harm than Good," in which he stated:

> [T]he large majority of PSA-discovered "cancers" would never cause any problem whatsoever if they went undetected . . . most of the men treated would have been just fine if they never knew about the cancer.

But when they're treated (whether with surgery, radiation, or chemo-therapy), the majority suffers really life-affecting effects, such as im-potence and/or incontinence. . . .

Contrast this to the comments of PSA discoverer Dr. Richard Ab-lin, who called it "a hugely expensive public health disaster," with accuracy "hardly better than a coin toss."[45]

On the very same day that Wilkes' op-ed article was published, the executive associate dean wrote a letter to the UCD Medical School associate dean for Curriculum stating that Wilkes would no longer continue as a doctoring instructor of record and the resources for a student exchange program that he had championed would be eliminated. The medical school dean was also informed that Wil-kes's "departmental space" would be reassigned. (The deans were referred to only by title in the official complaint.)[46]

In effect, Wilkes, a prominent professor commended by his peers and students for his contributions to academic excellence, was hav-ing his career dismantled because he wrote an op-ed piece voicing concern about the over-the-top promotion of PSA screening.

Wilkes dashed off an e-mail to the faculty members who had hosted the men's health event saying, "I am sorry if this caused your team unnecessary angst" and noting that his original article was substantially cut and edited in a way that might have created a more negative tone than the original version.[47] He even offered to take them to lunch and discuss educational opportunities and further clarify his position on the harms associated with PSA screening in healthy men. Wilkes's entreaties fell on deaf ears. The executive as-sociate dean added insult to injury by alleging that the timing of actions against Wilkes was purely coincidental. This ordeal dragged on until Wilkes finally appealed to the university's Committee on Academic Freedom and Responsibility (CAFR) and the Foundation for Individual Rights in Education (FIRE).

Both CAFR and FIRE responded forcefully. The two pas-sages below capture their respective arguments for Wilkes. Both CAFR and FIRE expressed indignation at the university's blatant intimidation of Wilkes, not to mention the insult to the First Amendment, a precept that should be especially dear to an institution of higher learning.

From CAFR, May 18, 2012:

> By unanimous assent CAFR has found that the faculty member's [Wilkes] academic freedom was violated by precipitous and inappropriate retaliatory statements of disciplinary sanction and legal action in the hours and days following the publication of a professional expert commentary perceived by some to be against University interests. Further, the violation persists such that the professor works in fear for his job and has to withhold his professional knowledge from students and society for fear of further retaliation.[48]

From FIRE, July 13, 2012:

> FIRE asks now that UC Davis formally withdraw the threats made against Michael Wilkes, publicly acknowledge its violation of his academic freedom, and reassure its faculty that they will not face retaliation for their expression.[49]

Two years after Wilkes's piece appeared in the *San Francisco Chronicle,* the University Senate's Representative Assembly, in a unanimous 52 to 0 vote, reprimanded administrators for the actions taken against Wilkes. The faculty panel also called for medical school leaders to apologize and "take concrete steps to prevent violations of the rights of academic freedom."[50]

In the end, that was all Wilkes wanted. He told me in a telephone interview that he regretted that his overall message about PSA screening might have been overshadowed by some of the op-ed's sharper tone. "There are better ways to deal with situations like this instead of being confrontational," Wilkes said. "The underpinning of academics is debate and discussion, not intimidation tactics."[51]

During our conversation, Wilkes did not identify the "sharper" tone that led to the University's censorious actions, but I'd lay odds that it came from the portion of his op-ed article in which he speculated that the university's motivation for offering the seminar *"just might have to do with money."* He explained that the practices of many urologists rely on PSA testing and the ensuing treatment and that urologists, as a group, are more favorably disposed toward the PSA "than almost any other doctors." He also noted that urologists are major contributors toward a "pro-PSA lobby."

Wilkes wondered if UCD's sponsorship of the men's health event had something to do with money. I don't wonder: I believe it certainly did. The AUA, using NFL star power, promoted mass PSA screening in men starting at age 40. It knew exactly how to tap into the male psyche and rev up the machismo machine. Create the male bonding experience—a band of brothers—and then hit them with the fear factor. It's a sure sell. Wilkes nailed it dead to rights. Then they tried to nail him for his audacity.

THE UNITED STATES IS THE MOST litigious country in the world. Our courts are jammed to capacity. Medical malpractice, with its potential for huge jury-awarded settlements, is a lucrative venue for aggressive lawyers. Reforming the tort laws that open the door for those settlements is a hotly debated topic in health care. (A tort is a civil wrong that causes somebody harm, as in malpractice cases.) Advocates of tort reform claim that by limiting the threat of frivolous lawsuits, the medical industry would be less apt to practice costly defensive medicine. On the reverse side of the coin, it is argued that the pressure of malpractice suits actually forces hospitals and doctors to be more efficient.

Let's now look at a case that illustrates one of the less talked about aspects that drives automatic PSA screening—fear of litigation. On July 19, 1999, Dr. Daniel Merenstein—a third-year resident (for legal reasons his institution requested anonymity)—saw a well-educated 53-year-old male patient who had never had a PSA test. Merenstein discussed the risks and benefits of PSA screening. The patient left without having a PSA test. Sometime later this patient saw another doctor who ordered a routine PSA test. His test number returned elevated. Subsequently, he was biopsied and diagnosed with advanced prostate cancer. The patient was forlorn; he felt that if his PSA had been tested on his initial visit with Merenstein, his prospects for survival would be better. As we have seen, the evidence does not support that theory. Nevertheless a lawsuit followed with the plaintiff's lawyer convincing a jury that evidence-based medicine warranted a $1 million judgment against Merenstein's residency program.[52]

Merenstein explained, "A major part of the plaintiff's case was that I did not practice the standard of care in the Commonwealth of Virginia. Four physicians testified that when they see male patients older than 50 years, they have no discussion with the patient about prostate cancer screening: they simply do the test."[53]

So much for shared-decision-making conversations.

Merenstein summed up how this episode changed the way he practiced medicine: "During that year before the trial, my patients became possible plaintiffs to me and I no longer discussed the risks and benefits of prostate cancer screening. I ordered more laboratory and radiological tests and simply referred more. My patients and I were the losers."[54] Such is the price of fear.

SIX

THE HIDDEN TRUTH

I am a 59-year-old white male, 8 months post-op. My cancer was found by accident. . . . I was enjoying life, sexually active . . . now, I work hard not to piss on myself when I exercise . . . and despite all the suction devices and Viagra . . . my life as a man is non-existent. . . . I really wonder if this is all I have to look forward to until I die.

—Anonymous, posted on MD Junction–
Prostate Cancer Support Group

What is manhood?

To say it is the opposite of womanhood certainly doesn't delineate the nuanced differences between the sexes. To an extent, manhood is a blurry demarcation in the psychophysical journey that begins at puberty. Most cultures mark that transition with some form of celebration, oftentimes religious, as in the Christian confirmation or the Jewish bar mitzvah. Indigenous cultures are known for some of the more hair-raising rites of passage designed to prepare young boys for the challenges of life. The Satere-Mawe tribe in the Amazon jungle uses the incredibly painful stings of bullet ants (so named because their sting feels like being shot with a .22-caliber bullet) to usher boys into manhood. At 13 years of age, Satere-Mawe boys must endure ten minutes of hell as they slip their hands into mesh gloves loaded with hundreds of bullet ants. The neurotoxic poison can leave a boy vomiting and in spasms for several days. This brutal rite of passage is repeated more than 20 times over the course of several months.[1] My own bar mitzvah had its uncomfortable moments, but nothing like that.

Manhood cannot be separated from virility, a term that is associated with a wide range of characteristics, such as vigor and health and procreation. *The Oxford English Dictionary* defines virility as "marked by strength of force."[2] Virility, however, is the most celebrated part of a man's sexuality. Greek and Roman mythology is rife with characters that embody male sexual power, like the oversexed god Pan, who gamboled in the wild mountains with a retinue of nymphs.[3] The absurdly oversized and perpetually erect phallus of the minor Greek god Priapus—from which the medical term *priapism* (an erection that fails to return to its flaccid state) is derived—is repeatedly frustrated by losing his erection just before the act, signaling one of the first cases of erectile dysfunction (ED). Even though he was a god, ED crippled his psyche.

Think how it must affect us poor mortals.

The interplay between sexual health and a man's overall sense of well-being is a very delicate balancing act that can be short-circuited by many factors. The quote from "Anonymous" at the beginning of the chapter echoes a common emotional thread binding together men who have had a radical prostatectomy. It's the feeling of lost manhood, which is not properly tackled in the larger conversation about PSA screening; that feeling gets lost in the mechanics of sex.

It is more than being able to get a successful erection. Too many people play down the sense of lost manhood and its downstream effects. Skip Lockwood, CEO of the megaprostate cancer advocacy organization ZERO, remarked that Dr. Otis Brawley of the American Cancer Society cared more about men's sex lives than about saving the men themselves, all because Brawley has become leery of PSA's clinical value. Lockwood's tone was shallow, condescending, and way off the mark—surprising for a man in his position.[4]

In 1999 I gave a presentation on prostate cancer for the support group Man to Man, hosted by the American Cancer Society. I was pointing out how the prostate industry rolled out well-known public figures to promote PSA screening. As an example, I held up a copy of a then popular cancer magazine called *InTouch*.[5] The issue pictured the late General Norman Schwarzkopf on its cover. During the interview he discussed his prostate cancer diagnosis and subsequent radical prostatectomy that left him with side effects that he was loath to delve into. He said that his cancer was slow growing and confined to the prostate. Asked about impotence issues, he snapped, "Nothing makes you more impotent than death. You've got to have your priorities!" He said that he was offered watchful waiting, but that approach wasn't in his makeup.[6]

Regarding my earlier point about manhood, Schwarzkopf related a telling anecdote. Several months after his radical prostatectomy, he was standing in the middle of the "raging Alagnak River in Alaska hooking a 50-pound king salmon." Just weeks later Stormin' Norman was on a big game safari in Tanzania where he encountered a Cape buffalo, considered among Africa's most dangerous game. "He charged, but I got him before he got me," Schwarzkopf told *InTouch*. "I needed that primeval experience to prove to myself that life goes on and life is good."[7]

To me, it sounds like the general suffered a major case of over-compensation for erectile dysfunction. Like millions of men before him, Schwarzkopf's radical prostatectomy left him feeling like he wasn't the man he used to be and for that personal shortcoming a poor buffalo minding his own business in sub-Saharan Africa was gunned down—another innocent victim of PSA screening. Think of it: if an imposing bearlike man who led an army into battle feels a loss of manhood from prostate surgery, imagine the crippling effect on less confident men.

THE SECOND OPINION

By the late 1990s PSA screening had become entrenched in medical practice. Such is the power of sophisticated marketing machines; the bigger their reach into society, the easier it is for people to believe they cannot live without a PSA test. Even though the PSA forces tried at every turn to shunt me to the outer most margins of science, I kept writing and publicly challenging PSA.

Then I got an opportunity to reach a wider audience.

In 2000 I wrote a commentary about PSA for the inaugural edition of *Lancet Oncology*.[8] It garnered attention and I was invited to give a seminar at Tarzana Medical Center near Los Angeles. It was a whirlwind trip filled with lectures. At a dinner-seminar of the UCLA Urology Journal Club, at which I was the surprise guest, Leonard Marks, a prominent urologist sitting at my table told me to shut up after I questioned the Prostate Cancer Foundation's chief science officer, Howard Soule, about the true altruistic motivation of his boss, billionaire prostate cancer survivor and advocate Michael Milken, who was first famous as a Wall Street felon. Although I was yet to be introduced, it was now obvious who the surprise guest was!

During the trip, I lunched with well-known radio host and ombudsman David Horowitz in Beverly Hills. I wanted airtime on his radio show to rouse public attention about the ongoing PSA tragedy. Unfortunately, Horowitz, who was an award-winning reporter during the Vietnam War, appeared gun-shy about his sponsors' reaction if he let me loose on the PSA industry. I'd won him over on the issue but he felt it was too radical an attack on mainstream medicine to chance. Instead, Horowitz agreed to let me use my 30-minute segment on the show to educate his audience on another subject I'd told him about—the female prostate. Yes, women have a prostate gland.[9]

A week after I appeared on Horowitz's show, I received a follow-up note from him, saying that his urologist, Alan Shapiro, MD, echoed my misgivings about PSA screening. Given that very few urologists supported my PSA stance out loud, Horowitz put us together. I met with Shapiro several times. He agreed with me that routine PSA screening had created a national health disaster, crippling millions of healthy men.

The problem we faced was how to get our message out in a way that would gather enough attention to break through the PSA misinformation barrier. Shapiro knew a journalist Andy Meisler, who wrote for the *Los Angeles Times*. Shapiro and Meisler came to Tucson and I gave them a brief presentation on PSA. Meisler was intrigued and we collaborated on an op-ed piece for the *LA Times*, which was rejected. Meisler knew famed *Washington Post* journalist Bob Woodward. He sent the piece to Woodward, who had no interest.

We decided to take the bull by the horns and formed a not-for-profit organization called the Cure Prostate Cancer Now Foundation. A wealthy patient of Shapiro's donated the seed money for the foundation. But we still needed an instrument to get the message about PSA screening into the public debate. We considered creating a newsletter, but ultimately decided that making a documentary would be the best way to grab the public's attention about the misuse of PSA screening for profit.

A young director-producer, Sheri Sussman, and Earl Lestz, former president of the Paramount Pictures Studio Group, who had contacts in Hollywood, took up the project. Brimming with enthusiasm, Sussman felt that, in addition to getting our message out on the misuse of PSA screening, the documentary's controversial subject matter would have a good chance of making some noise at independent film festivals such as Robert Redford's Sundance Film Festival. From there we could parlay the attention and pitch it to cable TV or a mainstream news outlet. After some skillful editing by Sussman, Wesley Tabayoyong II, and their associates, the documentary emerged as a forceful rendering of the PSA issue.

About 200 people viewed our premier of the documentary, *The Second Opinion*,[10] at Paramount Picture's Sherry Lansing Theatre on June 20, 2008. Many of the men in the audience were visibly upset, but the critics praised it. Here is a portion of a *Los Angeles Times* review by Susan Brink:

> There were groans in the audience, knowing nods of the head, a good number of men leaving auditorium seats in a rush to the bathroom, and wives giving a comforting rub to their spouses' arms at each intimate revelation in the documentary they were watching, "The Second Opinion." Many of these men . . . had more than a casual interest in prostate cancer. They've lived through its impossible choices and the

mutilating results of its treatment. Some of them were as sad, frustrated and angry as the men on the screen . . . that [the recognition about the harms associated with PSA] should make Richard Ablin happy. He's the guy who discovered the protein PSA back in 1970. "The PSA test is an absolute, total catastrophe," Ablin said after the screening.[11]

NOW I'LL INTRODUCE YOU to a diverse group of men who had their lives affected by PSA, beginning with a man you've already met, Dr. Alan Shapiro, one of the very few urologists during that earlier period who agreed with my struggle to shed light on the nightmare caused by PSA screening. All of these men appeared in *The Second Opinion*.

"The bottom line is that despite a marginal increase in surgical success, no man is ever the same after a radical prostatectomy, whether it's done as an open procedure or robotically," Shapiro said as we spoke about *The Second Opinion* at the premier.

In an interview, Shapiro said his personal turning point on the unnecessary harms caused by PSA screening was when a 50-year-old man came to his urology practice wearing a condom catheter—a flexible, condom-like sheath that fits over the penis and is attached to a tube that drains the urine into a urinary storage bag. "This relatively young guy had a radical prostatectomy, and now he couldn't get an erection or control his urine. He was crippled. I suddenly felt like that guy in the movie *Network,* screaming, 'I'm mad as hell and I'm not going to take this anymore.' I must do something about it!" Shapiro said.[12] This incident took place about five years before Shapiro and I decided to make our documentary.

The Second Opinion opens with a fairly young man lamenting the closeted nature of prostate health issues—PSA, biopsy, surgery, impotence. "It isn't the sort of thing men talk about when they're having a beer at the bar." As the credits roll, several men give brief impassioned messages, each one connected by a single acronym: PSA. Another 40-something man says, "They told me I might be a little incontinent and a little impotent." His facial language imparts a wry disbelief in what the word *little* would mean to his quality of life if he took his doctor's recommendation to have a radical prostatectomy. These are not actors; they are men and women who suffer degrading fortunes—most of them feel betrayed by our medical system.

Gene Light, a retired art director for Time Warner. At 75, Light's white hair and soft-spoken manner belies his zest for life. In 1991 the 53-year-old Light saw his doctor for a minor urinary tract infection. He was put on an antibiotic, which cleared it up. "The doctor had also taken a PSA test and informed me it was 9 ng/mL. I didn't even know what PSA was. A couple of weeks later I had another PSA test, which was 12. I just ignored it and went on with my happy life," Light said. But a year later when his PSA spiked to 19 his doctor insisted that he see a urologist for a biopsy. He did, and a week later the urologist called and told him he had prostate cancer. "When I heard 'cancer' it felt like I was in a falling elevator. For a month I was a basket case. I would go to a movie and tell my wife that it was probably the last movie I'll ever see."

Light's panic-stricken wife urged him to "just have it out." The urologist gave his shell-shocked patient two choices: radical prostatectomy or radiation. "I wish he had mentioned watchful waiting. But years after the surgery my wife asked if I could go to bed every night knowing there was a cancer in my prostate. Honestly, I couldn't," said Light.

He had a radical prostatectomy and while thankful that the incontinence was short-lived, the surgery left him unable to have sex with his wife. "Not that I was a stud," said Light with a sad smile, "but before the operation I had a sex life."

Although Light comes across as a likable, easy man to talk to, he does not shy away from the one thing that haunts him. "I've been impotent since my surgery and it really bothers me to no end. It's psychologically devastating. Nobody ever tells you, but after a radical prostatectomy you're never the same."

The words "never the same" ring with a grim finality and it takes a certain type of person to say them without sounding full of self-pity.

Light makes it clear that he lost something that will never be retrieved and it hurts. After a prostate cancer diagnosis, wives and lovers commonly reassure their man that all they want is for him to be alive. Light's alive, but not in the same way he was before the surgery.

Charles Alleyne, a soft-spoken African American man in his early 50s was diagnosed with prostate cancer when he was 46 years old. Turning back time, he remembered being distraught and confused; his terrified wife just wanted the cancer out. But his recollection of the decision-making process is blurred, giving the impression that his journey from a 5.1 PSA to the operating room was fast-tracked and impersonal. Alleyne's surgery left him with debilitating incontinence and impotence, subjects he admits are difficult for him to talk about.

At first, his eyes wander away when he says the word *impotence*. Surprisingly, there's no bitterness in his voice as he describes the post-op procedures he underwent to correct his side effects. "I'm still incontinent, and it makes everything I do tougher. I'm always worried I won't be able to find a bathroom if I'm out. I'm an avid cyclist, so I've had to curtail that a bit. But the impotence is terrible. I had a penile implant but it got infected so bad I had to have it redone. It's an inflatable pump device, which works. I've got it down to a science," said Alleyne. After a long pause, he added, "It's difficult, but it's just something you have to learn to live with." He confided that his urologist never suggested watchful waiting on his glide path from PSA to biopsy to the operating room.

There is no other way to frame it: Light and Alleyne were victims of the medical system and their road to victimhood began with a routine PSA test. It was disturbing to watch them relate their stories—they were permanently damaged, yet they refused to whine about surgeons carving out just enough of their manhood to leave them wondering forever whether it was worth it. They were so shocked by the word *cancer* that the details of their conversations with their doctors faded away. Studies show that men are more emotionally locked than women when discussing personal health issues. Thus, men like Light and Alleyne are more apt to blindly follow their doctor's orders. To witness the arrogant disdain surgeons have for the male body when they minimize the side effects of robotic radical prostatectomy, watch any number of online videos about the procedure.[13]

George Sugarman was a robust and genial man savoring the rewards of a good marriage that produced two successful children. Moving into early middle age, Sugarman carried himself like a man contented with the life he'd built for himself but still eager for more. His wife Susan, trim and pretty, said that in 2005, George went for a yearly physical and found that his PSA was elevated. Suddenly, their life frayed at the edges. His doctor repeated the PSA test; it came back at 4.1 ng/mL. He put Sugarman on an antibiotic, but the PSA remained slightly elevated. "My doctor suggested that I see a urologist, just to find out what was going on," said Sugarman. After a brief consult, the urologist strongly suggested a biopsy, just to be safe.

That's when reflexive anxiety set in.

"When I went for the biopsy, my PSA was 3.6 ng/mL. I had a trip with friends scheduled and I was on pins and needles waiting for the biopsy results," said Sugarman, adding, "I wasn't freaking out yet; I'm just not that kind of guy." But he couldn't leave for vacation with doubt hanging over his head. Remaining upbeat, he called for the results and remembers hearing only one word from the disembodied voice over the phone: cancer. "I was sitting on the edge of the bed telling my wife that I had prostate cancer. Then I started to cry," said Sugarman.

After he cleared his head he did what every man in his situation should do: he took a deep breath and started some levelheaded thinking. Prostate cancer is not an embolism that can kill instantly. "One part of me wanted to get the cancer out and be cured, but another part of me wanted to delay treatment," said Sugarman.

The urologist explained that he could have surgery or radiation. Sugarman had watched his mother's long death from cancer while on radiation and that experience soured him on that course of therapy. Sugarman asked the urologist about surgical side effects. "He said I'd be a little incontinent and a little impotent. I asked him to define little so I knew exactly what I was in for. He told me I would still be able to have an orgasm but would probably not be able to get an erection," said Sugarman, adding, "Not being able to have sex with my wife is not what I consider a little impotent."

Sugarman's wife, Susan, said, "The urologist called radical prostatectomy the 'gold standard.' He flat out told us that George was having surgery and everything would be fine. . . . I wanted George alive but I was also concerned about how a radical prostatectomy would affect him as a man."

Sugarman became a proactive patient. He packed up all his medical records and he and his wife went on a second-opinion tour of the best urologists in California, which culminated in a date to have a radical prostatectomy. "My wife was nervous, but by then we were in the 'just get it out' mode. A couple of days later a golf buddy of mine suggested I see this doctor friend of his. I had a surgery date but just to placate him I agreed," said Sugarman.

Having made the decision to have surgery, Sugarman was walking an emotional tightrope by agreeing to see another urologist. But the lesson here is that he was keeping an open mind about the most important decision of his life.

He saw the urologist his friend suggested.

Sugarman continued, "Interestingly, of all the big-shot urologists I'd seen, he was the only one who did a rectal exam [to palpate the prostate gland]. He didn't find anything abnormal. Then while looking through my records he smiled and said, 'I'm going to talk to you like a friend. There's a buzz going around that urologists are cutting out too many prostates. Out of the 12 core samples of your prostate there was cancer in only 1 percent of one sample. So 99 percent of your prostate is clear. You're a young guy, I think you should cancel the surgery.' He suggested that I wait a while and, if I want, have another biopsy."

Armed with renewed confidence, Sugarman confronted each of the previous urologists he'd seen and asked them, given his clinical report, if he was a candidate for watchful waiting. Each one said yes, leaving Sugarman chagrined that none of these doctors ever discussed watchful waiting as an option. He canceled his surgery and a year later he went for another biopsy to the same urologist who did the first—it came back cancer free. His wife Susan gushed with relief, but she quickly turned angry when recalling that her husband had been days away from an unnecessary, life-changing operation. "None of the other urologists we saw ever mentioned watchful waiting. I am not happy about that," Susan Sugarman said, leaving an unspoken question hanging in the air: Why?

The simple answer is money. Urologists make money by doing biopsies and cutting out prostates, not by watching. Thanks to her husband's moxie and his willingness to let reason win over fear, he dodged a bullet. However, despite Sugarman's brush with medical disaster, watching him and his wife, it's obvious that—although they're distressed that watchful waiting was never offered until seeing the friend of a friend's urologist—they seem emotionally detached and almost reluctant to connect money as a major reason George was being pressured into having a radical prostatectomy.

It is natural for patients to view their doctors through a lens that filters out unseemly human behavior such as avarice. In fact, Sugarman confided that he actually needed to build up his courage to seek other opinions, feeling that he was betraying his first urologist. Many of the other men in the documentary stated that they would follow their doctor's orders, without question. But should they?

A 2012 study published in *Health Affairs* sheds light on why many urologists use their white-coat power of persuasion and make decisions based on profit even when they are not in the best interests of their patients. The author, Jean M. Mitchell, used the perfect environment to observe urologists' behavior: self-referral of prostate cancer biopsies. Self-referral is when physicians order tests on a patient

198 THE GREAT PROSTATE HOAX

that are performed at a facility where they have a financial interest. As wrongheaded as it seems, federal law allows Medicare to reimburse this perversely incentivized practice.

Mitchell analyzed Medicare data from 36,261 biopsies and found that self-referring urologists billed Medicare for 4.3 more specimens per prostate biopsy than non–self-referring urologists—a whopping 72 percent difference. In short, Mitchell found that financial incentives prompt self-referring urologists to perform more biopsies on men who are very unlikely to have prostate cancer.[14] Another study on urologist self-referral, which was released in 2013 by the GAO, was even more damning. The GAO found that urologists who recently began referring prostate specimens to their own in-office labs *immediately* increased their pathology utilization by almost 60 percent.[15] The self-referral loophole is a hefty bill for the already beleaguered Medicare program, one that also exacts an exorbitant human toll.

The Second Opinion ends with a man in the shadows. Like someone in the witness-protection program, he asked that his interview be conducted in a room dimmed just enough to render him as an anonymous silhouette. He also requested that we use only his first name, Robert. In the summer of 2004 he received a call from his primary care doctor saying that his PSA had risen to 7 ng/mL. "I knew nothing about PSA. But the number caused enough alarm that a PhD friend of mine suggested I try this relatively new treatment called cryosurgery in which they freeze the prostate, killing any cancer cells. So I did," Robert said.

Robert was nearly 80 years old and this was his first trip to a hospital. He remembered the procedure being fairly easy to deal with. "But a couple of weeks later, while playing golf I began having extreme pain and lost control of my bladder. I had a catheter implanted but the symptoms went on for about six weeks," Robert said, adding, "Eventually I became so weak I couldn't walk without assistance." Robert choked back his emotions as he talked about seeing another physician for a second opinion, who immediately admitted him to the ER with a cataclysmic infection.

"The infection had already destroyed parts of my internal organs. The cryosurgery had perforated my bladder and bowel and created fistulas [abnormal connections between tissues, albeit a very rare serious AE with today's advanced cryotechnology]. To correct the fistulas, a surgeon removed a section of flesh from my leg and sewed it into my abdomen to separate the organs that were growing together," said Robert.

Robert had to have an eight-hour-long surgery to save his bladder, colon, and rectum. "They patched me up as well as they could. After surgery I no longer needed a colostomy or catheter, which I was thankful for. Of course I'm totally incontinent and impotent," he said, and then shaking his head he added, "I eventually had my prostate removed, which perhaps I should have done first . . . or maybe at 78 years old I shouldn't have done anything. This really changed my life," said Robert, with quiet dignity as he faded to black.

With implausible recklessness, Robert's primary care doctor set off a false alarm by ordering a PSA test for Robert, an elderly man. It was an egregious error. More than 80 percent of all men his age already have prostate cancer and 97 percent of those men will die of another cause. Robert was healthy and enjoying his life, so why submit him to procedures that would ultimately degrade his quality of life? They should have left Robert alone so he could wind down his life's journey playing golf with friends. What was done to him, irrespective of any treatment, was beyond malpractice—it was criminal.

In paraphrasing the comments of Raymond B. Nagle, MD, PhD, a physician-scientist at the University of Arizona specializing in pathology and noted for his work on prostate cancer, and the other physician in the documentary: the PSA test is a bad test, we truly need a better test, and as most urologists are surgeons, surgeons are trained to cut.

In the end, *The Second Opinion* was a noteworthy documentary, the first film to critically look at the human effect of the PSA test. We hired a publicist and launched a strategic marketing plan, doing a lot of the legwork ourselves. We approached TV networks and radio stations. But debunking the PSA test stepped on the toes of too many sponsors, such as Pfizer, which at the time was heavily promoting its blockbuster ED drug Viagra.

I suspect that the pro-PSA screening environment in the early 2000s, awash with celebrity advocates, also dampened the media's eagerness to give me a platform to challenge the received wisdom. Getting airtime on a credible stage was a Sisyphean battle. It reminded me of the famous scene from the military drama *A Few Good Men* when the character played by Tom Cruise shouted that he wanted the truth, and the marine played by Jack Nicholson shouted back, "You can't handle the truth!" Most people simply did not want to handle the truth about PSA. Men didn't want the truth—they wanted a test that was going to save them from dying of prostate cancer.

Money can also create a convenient state of denial. I've met prominent leaders in biotech companies, and after explaining why the PSA test does not detect cancer, the typical reaction was vague interest. More telling was the universal gesture for money, rubbing their thumb and index finger. Or the brazenly honest reply: "We're just making too much money to rock the boat."

I asked a well-known public health researcher, Timothy Wilt, MD, MPH, for his thoughts on why so many men blindly follow their doctor's recommendation on PSA tests that often lead to unnecessary treatments. Wilt, a primary care doctor, observed, "Early detection and screening are embedded in medical culture, also in the patient population. It just seems to make too much sense to argue against. Find something bad when it's small and cut it out before it gets big. Of course that's not always the case, especially in prostate cancer." Asked how he approaches PSA, he said, "I recommend against PSA testing and only order a test if my patient adamantly requests it. Even then, I discuss the potential harms associated with PSA test," Wilt said.[16]

Now I want to introduce a friend of mine, Alvin "Al" Cox: to my mind he exemplifies the educated health care consumer. He didn't blindly follow his doctor's advice: instead, he did his own risk assessment after receiving an elevated PSA.

Al Cox has a passing resemblance to Charlton Heston—a quiet resolve emphasized by pale blue eyes that always meet yours halfway during conversation. His sun-and-wind-burnished face is a permanent reminder of his earlier life—sailing the high seas from San Diego to Bora Bora to Singapore and beyond in a 36-foot sailboat named *Seaforth*. Cox, a licensed general contractor by the age of 25, made a fortune building apartments and medical buildings in downtown San Diego. He retired in 1976 and, with his wife, Joan, sailed out of San Diego Bay, plying the world's oceans and far-flung ports-of-call for 38 years. As a man who gets seasick in a bathtub, I cannot imagine the storms that Cox faced during his time at sea. I mention his life as an itinerant sailor simply because the self-reliance and critical-thinking skills needed for survival on the open ocean were used during another challenge: being diagnosed with prostate cancer.

Recently, I talked with Cox in the lobby of the Hyatt Regency Hotel in San Diego. He told me, "In 1994, after a slightly elevated PSA test, I had a biopsy and was diagnosed with prostate cancer. I was as frightened as any other man hearing the word 'cancer.' My Gleason score was 6, which put me in the gray zone concerning the next move," Cox told me, adding, "But my urologist told me to take a couple of weeks to digest it all and then I needed to have my prostate gland removed."[17]

If radical prostatectomy was next, Cox wanted to be sure that he had the best surgeon possible. His research led him to Johns Hopkins Medical Institution and Patrick C. Walsh, MD, the father of the so-called nerve-sparing radical prostatectomy. But there was a three-month-long wait to see the famous surgeon, so Cox filled the time by seeing four other urologists. "One told me, 'You don't have three months to wait, you have a killer inside of you that needs to get right out.' Despite the urgent warning of that one urologist, I decided to wait to see Dr. Walsh, and do my own research on prostate cancer and in the interim, I sent Dr. Walsh a letter with a list of questions," said Cox.

He collected a data bank of literature from prostate cancer support groups and from library searches. "The stack of data was about three feet high. I began critically analyzing all the information, looking at the pros and cons of treatment. And the data indicated that my life expectancy would be about the same with or without treatment. Moreover, less than 3 percent of men with prostate cancer will die [of the disease]," said Cox. He took his research deeper. At that time, it was being widely reported that 44,000 American men per year were dying of prostate cancer. "So I went to several medical libraries and pored over the prostate cancer mortality data going back to 1950, a year in which 12,500 men died of prostate cancer." That number increased steadily until the advent of the PSA test, then it skyrocketed to the 44,000 deaths.

The huge increase in prostate cancer deaths left him perplexed. In 1997 Cox spoke with Benjamin F. Hankey, ScD, director of NCI's Surveillance Epidemiology and End Results (SEER), the government's massive data bank of disease outcomes. Hankey explained that prostate cancer deaths in older men are associated with a host of competing medical conditions such as heart disease and diabetes, which leads to errors in certification (attribution) of death. Cox dug deeper, accessing mortality data from the Centers for Disease Control (CDC) database. He found that in 1997 there were 32,891 deaths attributed to prostate cancer versus 47,063 deaths that mentioned prostate cancer on the death certificate.[18] Therefore, Cox speculated that the higher *nonspecific* attribution of prostate cancer had been used to elevate the mortality numbers.

Meanwhile, Cox never received a reply from Walsh regarding his questions. "I finally telephoned Walsh," Cox said. "I was speaking to his assistant and I overheard her say, 'It's Mr. Cox calling about the answers to his questions.' Then I heard Dr. Walsh reply in the background, 'Tell Mr. Cox we do not need him as a patient.' I abruptly canceled my appointment."

Cox's tenacious research gathered steam. "I began making mortality graphs and mailing them out to people and organizations," he said. He wanted to know everything about PSA and his search led to me. I remember his out-of-the-blue call one night. Al was very polite but blunt, saying, "Dr. Ablin, according to my research the PSA test is leading men to their death." There was a stunned pause before I said, "I couldn't agree with you more, Mr. Cox." One conversation led to another that formed a casual alliance in which we would exchange information about prostate cancer, which in turn Cox would use as a conduit to all the top people and organizations in the field.

Armed with his own data bank, Cox spent five years trying to get the truth about PSA out to the nation, working with cancer organization executives and media people such as ABC News anchor Peter Jennings and *New York Times* journalist Larry Katzenstein. Cox feels that he made a difference but to his dismay, despite the overwhelming amount of data showing that the harms of PSA screening heavily outweigh potential benefits, the prostate cancer industry, based largely on PSA testing, is still flourishing.

Ironically, John Blum, MD, the urologist who had performed Cox's biopsy—a mutual yacht club member and avid sailor—was diagnosed with prostate cancer himself, two months after Cox's diagnosis. Knowing Blum somewhat casually from the club, Cox sent him his prostate cancer data, showing him why he had decided against surgery. "He was impressed by the evidence I'd accumulated, but he said, 'Al, the data you sent me is scary, it does give me pause, but I'm a urologist who's been taking out prostates for the past 30 years. I have no choice.'"

Cox said that his urologist friend had a radical prostatectomy resulting in such severe urinary incontinence that he was re-operated on to have a stent implanted. "The stent got infected and he had to go in for what turned out to be three more implants, ending in such powerful infection that it destroyed his equilibrium. A man that was an accomplished sailor ended up walking with two canes. He died two years later of an aneurism," said Cox.

At 75, Al Cox plays a good game of tennis and still enjoys the vigorous challenge of blue-water sailing.

IN 2004, MY EFFORTS SEEMED to bear fruit as I caught the interest of ABC's chief investigative journalist, Brian Ross. An acquaintance of Larry Kelly (of the Glynn & Mercep law firm, mentioned in chapter

5), Ross was interested in the qui tam action concerning the use of PSA screening. We filmed a segment for one of his upcoming reports. I felt very confident that I'd delivered a cogent message about PSA, answering all of Ross's questions and rebutting the claims that PSA saved men's lives. Most importantly, I made a solid case that routine PSA screening in healthy men was nothing short of a national health disaster. At last, I was given the chance to explain the truth about PSA screening to the public at large. Then, about two months later, while in Tokyo for a research conference, I received a cable indicating ABC was most likely killing the segment. I was crestfallen. Numb. Angry. From what information I was given by Kelly on my return to the United States, ABC, in doing its due-diligence review of the segment, had spoken with William J. Catalona and Roswell Park. I don't know exactly what was said, but the show was abruptly canceled.

Even more upsetting was the fact that the ABC show was not about my discovering PSA but about its widespread misuse. And, ironically, it all began at Roswell Park. They were just protecting their franchise, but of course ABC didn't know that.

Looking back, my biggest regret is that men like Robert didn't have their say. He's not a prostate cancer survivor—he's a victim and he needed someone to tell him that in his particular circumstances, what was done to him was wrong.

SEVEN

IT'S 112 DEGREES
IN TUCSON

From: *[Name Removed for Confidentiality]*
Subject: *PSA Test*
Date: *Oct 3, 2012 9:49 AM*
Dear Dr. Ablin:

Thank you for your work in the area of dispelling PSA myths. I only wish I would have been informed on this topic 6 months ago before my doctor randomly added the PSA test to my physical. I'm on the "prostate biopsy train" and my life feels like it's spinning out of control. . . . I am only 43 years old with no history of disease in my family, although I have suffered from prostatitis. . . . I often have panic attacks and wake up from nightmares because I'm confused and angry that this has been dropped in my lap. . . . Thank you again for fighting the good fight in the highly contentious area of health care.

—One of thousands of e-mails I have
received over the years

As you turn the last page of this book, my hope is that, first and foremost, it has been a compelling read, one that has left you feeling more fully informed. Although the purpose of the book—exposing abuse of power and the profit-over-patient ethos that caused the PSA public health disaster—is fairly straightforward, the story is filled with complexities. I've tried to show the forest in spite of the trees. While writing the book, I have often reflected on my discovery of PSA in 1970, and I am left wondering how three letters and a tiny gland could have caused so much trouble.

In the middle of the 1900s an Austrian economist named Joseph Schumpeter coined the term *creative destruction* to describe a type of transformation in which a status quo is replaced by radical innovation.[1] For millennia medicine advanced in crude increments, mostly based on basic observation and pure guesswork. The first creative destruction in medicine occurred in the early 1830s when a few leading physicians publicly stated that most of the medical treatments being used at the time were not only ineffective, but that they did more harm than good.[2] I can only imagine the blowback these brave doctors faced for having the temerity to challenge the medical establishment.

Almost 200 hundred years later, you have repeatedly read the same "more harm than good" phrase on the pages of this book to describe routine PSA screening. Medicine has a long history of providing cover for procedures that have no benefit for patients. In 1876 Harvard professor Edward Clarke reviewed studies that showed that patients with typhoid fever could recover by themselves, without medical intervention, and often did far better than those who received the treatments that were popular at the time.[3] But the concept that sometimes doing less or even nothing is better for patients runs contrary to the medical philosophy of treating everything with something. This entrenched doctor-patient mindset has buttressed the prostate cancer industry's exploitation of PSA and has had a chilling effect on my public call to end routine screening of healthy men.

My ultimate goal in writing this book is to do what had hitherto seemed impossible: make Washington accountable for the grievous public health disaster caused by the unfettered promotion of PSA screening and hopefully prevent another similar episode in American health care. As individuals, we can be optimistic about our prospects for health, happiness, and prosperity. But, when it comes to the government, the feeling of optimism is decidedly different. Most polls indicate that Americans suffer a malaise of extreme pessimism about our federal government's ability to function efficiently and scrupulously. My hope is that the creative destruction of the PSA-driven model in prostate health will restrain the government-sanctioned deployment of tests before there is solid evidence to justify their clinical value.

ON MARCH 10, 2010, I published an op-ed piece in the *New York Times,* "The Great Prostate Mistake." In the piece, I expressed my frustration with policy makers who have their collective heads buried in the sand about PSA screening:

> The test's popularity has led to a hugely expensive public health disaster. It's an issue I am painfully familiar with—I discovered P.S.A. in 1970. As Congress searches for ways to cut costs in our health care system, a significant savings could come from changing the way the antigen is used to screen for prostate cancer. . . . I never dreamed that my discovery four decades ago would lead to such a profit-driven public health disaster. The medical community must confront reality and stop the inappropriate use of PSA screening. Doing so would save billions of dollars and rescue millions of men from unnecessary, debilitating treatments.[4]

The article excited a firestorm of reaction, particularly from the urological community and patient advocates. Several power brokers in the prostate cancer industry contacted the *Times* in an attempt to discredit me. I responded with a mountain of irrefutable data that was more than satisfactory for the *Times.* The editor I worked with said that "The Great Prostate Mistake" was one of the most widely read op-ed pieces on the *Times*'s website in the paper's recent history. I received hundreds of e-mails, innumerable letters via the post, and many telephone calls. A few were scathing retorts, calling me a murderer of men for recommending against population PSA testing. In fact two or three callers inquired how much the Obama administration was paying me to discourage medical testing in the elderly. However, most of the letters expressed thanks for shedding light on this continuing conundrum, including the one quoted at the opening of this chapter. That patient described in stark terms the psychological torture of being in the limbo land between PSA tests. I found it heartbreaking when he spoke about his life "spinning out of control," with panic attacks, nightmares, confusion, and anger.

It does not have to be that way.

A WOLF IN SHEEP'S CLOTHING

As discussed in an earlier chapter, in 2013 the AUA backed off its aggressive PSA stance. But this move toward moderation was simply a political smokescreen providing cover for emerging PSA replacement technologies. Make no mistake: although these next-generation PSA tests are sophisticated and the high-powered pitchmen behind them convincing, they are not prostate cancer-specific and have limited clinical relevance at best. So let's look at an example of how these new early-detection tests are currently being marketed by using heavyweights in prostate cancer.

E. David Crawford, MD, is an internationally recognized prostate cancer expert. Like most high-profile urologists, Crawford is a paid consultant for several large pharmaceutical companies and the lead researcher on many industry-funded clinical trials. Having a paid powerhouse urologist like Crawford running the trial also boosts the chance of FDA approval.

Among his various activities, Crawford is the chairman of the Prostate Conditions Education Council (PCEC). According to its website, the PCEC organizes hundreds of free or low-cost screening sites for men across the country each year during Prostate Cancer Awareness Month, which has resulted in nearly 5 million men being provided with PSA tests.[5] And Crawford is just one of many promoters, herding millions more men onto the PSA-testing train. So how did he react to the new PSA-light guidelines that were released on May 3, 2013? This is what Crawford had to say:

> The PCEC applauds the American Urological Association for its diligent work on their new prostate cancer clinical practice guidelines announced today and its recognition that, as medicine continues to evolve, so must the protocols for the disease. We look forward to continuing the discussion around the best practices for the diagnosis and treatment of prostate cancer.[6]

Several days after the AUA released its new guidelines, the PCEC held an industry clinical update presentation at the annual AUA annual meeting, "Understanding How New Biomarkers Will Assist the Diagnosis and Prognosis for Prostate Cancer." Crawford led the presentation, ushering in a new early detection test called ConfirmMDx, made by MDxHealth. The company's press release even boasted that its test outperformed PSA in prostate cancer detection and helped urologists rule out prostate cancer-free men from unnecessary repeat biopsies.[7]

During an interview at the conference, Crawford explained that he was "very excited" about ConfirmMDx, which, he said, can be used to reexamine tissue from a previous negative biopsy to identify changes in the cells that might suggest the need for another biopsy.[8]

Crawford used a case history to demonstrate the value of this new test. A 46-year-old man went for a consult because his PSA was elevated to 9 ng/mL. He'd had a prior negative biopsy. Several months before, a severe urinary infection landed him in the hospital where he was treated with antibiotics and released. In the interim period, his PSA fell from 13 to 9, but he was still anxious and went to see Crawford.

> Except for some urinary symptoms, the patient seemed healthy, Crawford reported. His sexual function was normal. His prostate appeared to be normal, too, based upon a rectal exam. His PSA had declined to 6.1. But, as a precaution, twelve tissue samples from his previous

biopsies were retested using ConfirmMDx. The test showed a "positive" result in three of the samples. The man was then re-biopsied
and three cores showed Gleason scores of six. The patient then had a
radical prostatectomy.[9]

Crawford went on to state, "Regardless of one's opinion on
mass screening, most would agree that detection and treatment in a
healthy 46-year old man would be beneficial." One problem with a
biopsy, Crawford explained, is that it samples "less than 1 percent
of the gland."

"I've seen men biopsied more than a dozen times to follow up
steadily rising PSA levels until a cancer was found . . . [T]here is a lot
of hit and miss . . ." As a result, Crawford says, some physicians take
"a 'drill more holes, find more oil' approach."[10]

Let's consider the unnamed urologist to whom Crawford referred, who performed more than 12 biopsies on one patient; if that
urologist charged $2,000 a biopsy, he presumably pocketed about
$25,000. If, after using the "drill more holes, find more oil" ap-
proach, he finally found some cancer, he may have earned himself a
$20,000 payday for a radical prostatectomy. Add up the office visits
and prescriptions and this urologist may have pocketed well more
than $50,000 from one man.

I'm more than a little dubious that, as Crawford said, "most
would agree" with how this healthy 46-year-old man was treated.
For one, his PSA had declined to 6.1 when he saw Crawford.

Recall my interview with one of the world's most highly regarded
pathologists, Jonathan Oppenheimer, MD, in chapter 3. "By calling
the 3 + 3 = 6 Gleason score 'cancer' pathologists are doing a disservice to patients, scaring them into having conditions treated that
will not harm them."[11] Oppenheimer is in a growing camp of doctors
that believe we need a new name for any finding that is scored Gleason 6 or below. As he mentioned, take away the C-word and men
will be far less susceptible to making fear-driven decisions.

Robert Weiss, MD, writing on the website CancerNetwork, had
severe reservations about Crawford's case study:

Will someone explain to me why a patient coming out of a urinary infection (perhaps a harder to treat prostate infection) and having just undergone a biopsy (negative), and whose PSA was monotonically— falling from 13 to 9.0 to 6.1—was not sent home *to enjoy his life without further insult or testing?* [Emphasis added.][12]

In light of the patient's prior urinary infection, which might have been responsible for raising his PSA, Weiss also questioned the advisability of the original biopsy before determining whether additional antibiotics would bring down the PSA numbers.

Weiss's spirited assessment speaks volumes about the continuing problem that overshadows the future of men's prostate health: the urology and oncology community, the device makers, and those who profit from the ancillary treatments and services associated with prostate cancer will find very creative ways to keep the early-detection-to-treatment train steaming along. This is the classic hammer looking for nails and Crawford typifies the hammer.

MISTAKEN KINDNESS

Monetary gain aside, simple human nature has also contributed mightily to the medical community's stubborn refusal to acknowledge the disaster of PSA screening. Self-aggrandizement, or more simply the need to be relevant, is a compelling force in humanity. As a rule of thumb, the more powerful the person, the greater the need to protect whatever it is that gives that person relevance. As Francis Fukuyama pointed out in his excellent book, *The End of History and the Last Man,* "The desire for recognition sounds like a strange and somewhat artificial concept, the more so when it is said to be the primary motor driving human history."[13] Our medical history is filled with men who refused, in the face of evidence, to change their course even when it was proven wrong. This type of ego-driven conviction has led medicine into its darkest corners.

William Stewart Halsted was a famous surgeon whose name became the symbol of radical surgery. Halsted began his surgical career in the mid-1870s, a time when bloodletting, cupping, leeching, and surgical purging were standard medical practices. A trip to Europe proved fortuitous, as it was just the time when cancer surgery was beginning to surface in operating theaters. Halstead returned from Europe and began performing breast cancer surgeries with near superhuman energy. At the time, his addiction to cocaine and morphine was a well-kept secret. Halsted's surgical prowess improved, but he was vexed to distraction by the recurrence of cancer, usually reappearing at the margins where his scalpel had ceased cutting away the tissue.

An English surgeon named Charles Moore hypothesized, "Mammary cancer requires the careful extirpation of the entire organ. Local recurrence of cancer after operations is due to the continuous growth of fragments of the principal tumor."[14] The central conclusion was that surgeons were letting mistaken kindness for women prevent their scalpels from doing what was needed: radical removal of as much tissue as possible. Halsted and his surgical sycophants sliced away whole sections of the female anatomy, leaving women horribly disfigured. He vigorously promoted the Halsted radical mastectomy at medical conferences across the country. A doctor named George Crile, an outspoken critic of Halsted, pointed out that "if the breast cancer was so advanced that one had to get rid of the tumor, then it had already spread through the system,"[15] obviously rendering the radical operation futile. In essence, Crile told Halsted that he had conviction but no proof that his surgery benefited women. And, as we've seen, the human consequences of medicine running ahead of proof are devastating.

Halsted's reaction to this attack should resonate with readers of this book. He said, "It is especially true of mammary cancer that the surgeon interested in furnishing the best statistics may in perfectly honorable ways provide them."[16] Imagine that. Halsted was so caught up in the narrative of his own fame that he failed to see the gaping ethical breech in his statement. To him, supplying your own favorable evidence to bolster your position was perfectly above board. Although Halsted never proved that more surgery translated into better therapy, generations of surgeons kept the mutilating practice alive. Then a doctor named Bernard Fisher proved that the Halsted radical mastectomy was no more effective than lumpectomy (a limited surgical procedure that just removes the tumor and preserves the breast), which is followed in some cases with radiation therapy.

Fisher wrote that "he was willing to have faith in divine wisdom, but not in Halsted as divine wisdom."[17] He also said, "In God we trust, all others must have data."[18] However, it took him and his colleagues about a decade to finally change the breast cancer surgical paradigm. Unfortunately, hundreds of thousands of women had already undergone unnecessary radical mastectomies. What's important about Halsted, other than an interesting medical story, is that he and generations of doctors following him surgically mutilated women despite having no hard evidence that radical mastectomy had clinical benefit. In fairness, many earlier surgeons truly believed that more is better and that the radical mastectomy approach led to cure. But after the evidence showing that radical mastectomy should be replaced with lumpectomy, the surgical community circled the wagons and went into resistance mode. That's similar to what we've seen in the prostate cancer community's refusal, despite the evidence, to halt routine PSA screening.

The radical mastectomy is rarely if ever, performed today—an entire culture of breast cancer surgeons slowly collapsed along with that paradigm change. I foresee the radical prostatectomy sharing the same fate as the radical mastectomy. As you read in chapter 6, the trial led by Dr. Timothy Wilt followed two groups of men who were diagnosed with localized prostate cancer for 12 years. One group had radical prostatectomies and the other group was simply observed (active surveillance). Wilt found that the men who had radical prostatectomy did not significantly reduce their chance of dying compared with the group of men who had no treatment. But, as with the Halsted radical mastectomy, despite no evidence that radical prostatectomy extends men's lives, prostate cancer surgeons will not go down without a long and bitter fight.

THE DOCTOR AND THE C-WORD

My colleague and friend Charlie L. Bennett, MD, PhD, MPP, is a nationally regarded medical oncologist and hematologist specializing in prostate cancer. Bennett, who's also an authority on medication safety, founded the consortium RADAR (Research on Adverse Drug Events and Reports), which to date has reported potentially deadly side effects associated with about 50 drugs. "So far we're 50 for 50 in identifying potentially fatal drug reactions," Bennett told me during a recent visit to the Arizona Cancer Center in Tucson.[19] "And the companies we've looked at all have multibillion-dollar revenues. We believe our work has saved more than 100,000 lives and $10 billion."[20]

Dr. Bennett has an investigative journalist's nose for medical news and an inquisitive mind that constantly searches out interesting stories in the world of oncology. At the age of 50, he became an interesting story himself when he stepped aboard the PSA train for the first time.[21] His PSA level was 1.5 ng/mL, which he felt was not alarming but it still caused concern. He had it checked again a year later—it had risen to 2.5 ng/mL. He met with a urologist who was a faculty colleague of his at the Robert H. Lurie Comprehensive Cancer Center Feinberg School of Medicine, Northwestern University. "I asked to have a biopsy which was performed about 6 weeks later. Naturally, I was anxious. I had treated hundreds of men with prostate cancer, and had seen thousands of biopsy slides. But this time it was me. I kept running different scenarios through my head," Bennett said.

A few days later he called the pathologist, another colleague, and was told the slides were ready. The pathologist even invited Bennett down to the lab to read them himself. Bennett bolted down the staircase and sat at the microscope table with his friend peering at a slide that, like a crystal ball, was a window into his future.

There it was, staring him in the face: his prostate cancer cells on a glass slide.

Now what?

The cancer was a Gleason score 3 + 3 = 6, evident in only 1 of 12 core samples. Just 5 percent of Bennett's prostate gland had cancer cells and there was no evidence that the cancer had spread to the lymph nodes or the seminal vesicles (a set of tube-like glands that produces the fluid that ultimately becomes semen). After the initial shock, Bennett cleared his head and took stock of the situation. He and the pathologist discussed the various treatment options, reviewing those from the leading medical, surgical, and radiation oncologists. After weighing the pros and cons of each treatment, Bennett chose to have a radical prostatectomy.

Bennett made an appointment to see a nationally recognized leader in prostate cancer surgery. After a lengthy consultation, he came away feeling that having a prostatectomy performed by one of the country's top surgeons would give him the best chance not only for a cure, but with very low risk of sexual, bladder, and bowel dysfunction. Even still, he was anxious, knowing that all surgeries carry risk. For one, he was an avid runner and he was concerned that the radical prostatectomy might render his daily five-mile jog a thing of the past. His surgeon assured him that after the usual post-op recuperation he could resume his routine.

Bennett had the radical prostatectomy. He went into the operating room with a nervously upbeat frame of mind. "Right after the surgery I knew there was a problem. My left arm and leg were weak; the two sides of my body felt different," he said. The exact nerve damage done to his body was never diagnosed, but it seems to have been permanent. Although radical prostatectomy is one of the most common surgeries, there is nothing common about the challenges faced in doing one. Here's an excerpt about radical prostatectomy from *Prostate Cancer UPDATE,* the newsletter of Johns Hopkins, one of the country's top university hospitals:

> As surgical procedures go, radical prostatectomy is one of the most delicate, intricate, and flat-out difficult to perform correctly. Proof of this can be found in the widely varying rates of success of surgeons at hospitals throughout the world—not simply in controlling cancer, but in preserving a man's quality of life in two major areas: urinary continence and sexual potency.[22]

To this day, Bennett is cancer free, but his daily five-mile run is no longer possible. If he had to do it all over again, Bennett said that he would not have had a radical prostatectomy—instead he would have opted for active surveillance.

It's worth noting that Charlie Bennett's nationally renowned surgeon is a doctor all too familiar to the readers of this book: William J. Catalona.

What's most instructive about Bennett's case is that you will not find a more informed patient. He's a recognized oncologist-hematologist and a health policy expert and he has treated prostate cancer patients for almost 30 years. Yet, as informed as he is, once he saw his PSA began to rise, there was an involuntary mental shift created by an array of internal forces, all set in motion by the fear of cancer. Given that, how can we expect most men, some of whom don't even know what a prostate gland is, to have a meaningful, shared-decision-making conversation about PSA screening during a routine office visit with their primary care doctor?

I asked Allan S. Brett, MD—a well-known internist with special interests in medical ethics and shared decision making—we co-authored a recent Perspective about the latter in the *New England Journal of Medicine*[23]—if he thought that the new AUA guidelines would affect the conversation in the doctor's office about PSA testing. He responded:

> Not really. It is a tough thing to boil all the potential benefits against the known harms associated with PSA testing into a conversation that a broad spectrum of men will understand and use to make a decision that has significant consequences. There's also the doctor's mentality that it's better to do something than nothing. For instance, in the VA hospital down here, they are routinely PSA testing elderly men who are very sick. I asked them why this practice persisted, one that obviously had no health benefits for these patients. The simple answer I got was that checking the PSA test order box was more or less an automatic response with the staff.[24]

In the more-is-better medical ethos that has long guided our health system, the VA staff is absolved from the guilt of over-treatment. However, giving an old sick man a PSA test that could lead to unnecessary procedures is an elusive form of malpractice conducted across the country.

LIES, DAMNED LIES, AND STATISTICS

First, whenever one talks about statistics, it's a good thing to couch the discussion in the wry phrase Mark Twain popularized in 1906 with the publication of *Chapters from My Autobiography*. Twain wrote, "Figures often beguile me, particularly when I have the arranging of them myself." He also made popular the phrase used to describe the convincing power of statistics to bolster one's argument: "There are three kinds of lies: lies, damned lies, and statistics."[25] Mark Twain was a beloved contrarian with an overly cynical view of the workings of the world. But he was correct when he said that statistics could be powerful, especially for the one arranging the numbers.

As I've mentioned, prostate cancer is a disease of age; the average age of diagnosis is about 67 and about half of all men in their 50s have prostate cancer. Each year about 240,000 men in the United States will be diagnosed with prostate cancer. However, of all the men diagnosed each year with prostate cancer, their lifetime risk of death from the disease is only 3 percent, which means, of course, that a man has a 97 percent chance of surviving a diagnosis of prostate cancer whether he receives treatment or not.

But what do statistics signify for the readers of this book? For one, proponents of routine PSA screening have hung their hat on a couple of statistical arguments they contend prove that screening catches cancers early when they are still treatable, thus saving men's lives and reducing the incidence of metastasis on diagnosis from the pre- versus post-PSA eras. The recent trial most often cited by PSA advocates is called the Göteborg (Sweden) study[26]—one of several

trials conducted in Europe and reported under the umbrella name
the European Randomized Study of Screening for Prostate Cancer
(ERSPC).[27] With harm from overdiagnosis at 30 to 100 times the
estimated benefit,[28] resulting in less than 0.1 percent (1 of 1,000
screened) reduction in prostate mortality over ten years[29] and with
over two decades of PSA screening, one cannot help but wonder
what cost we are willing to pay for such a small benefit.

However, studies that are conducted and aggregated at multiple sites across the globe suffer a mashup of data that oftentimes
adds more confusion than clarity. I asked Roger Chou, MD, MPH,
a prominent doctor and public health researcher to comment on the
Göteborg study's allure with PSA advocates. Chou, who was a lead
researcher for the US Preventive Services Task Force, said, "Using
Göteborg to represent benefits of prostate cancer screening really
seems like cherry picking as it is not truly an independent study with
most of its patients included in the ERSPC and especially since there
is nothing about the methods used in the Göteborg arm to explain
why its results were so much better."[30] In regard to the ERSPC trial
as a whole, it is important to appreciate that only 2 of 7 centers included in the trial had positive effects on mortality (Göteborg and
the Netherlands), which means 5 of 7 did not. And, the further report out of Göteborg after 14 versus 9 years in the ERSPC with a
high risk reduction represented an extended follow up of a selected
group of patients.[31] For the sake of completeness, the ERSCP reported a follow up at 11 years (of their core group of men 55 to 69
years of age)[32] that showed a 29 versus 20 percent reduction in death
from prostate cancer, but *no* effect on all-cause mortality. Moreover,
76 percent of the men were biopsied because of an elevated PSA, but
no cancer was found—they were false positives. Equally important,
any marginal benefit of PSA screening was overshadowed by the loss
of quality of life due to the long-term effects of the treatments.[33]

More important, when all is said and done, after reviewing the
most current data, the task force found that, at best, of the 1 in every 1,000 men given the PSA test may avoid death as a result of the
screening.[34]

In fact, PSA testing leads to gross overdiagnosis that can be creatively used to produce favorable outcomes. For example, when routine PSA screening exploded onto the scene in the late 1980s, the incidence of detected prostate cancer skyrocketed. This dramatic increase generated what's called lead-time bias, which simply means that earlier diagnoses artificially inflate the survival statistics because they extend the time to death. Troubled that the misreporting of prostate cancer survival rates would lead to an increased use of PSA testing, professors Gerd Gigerenzer and Odette Wegwarth of the Max Planck Institute in Berlin published an insightful paper in the *British Medical Journal,* "Five-Year Survival Rates Can Mislead." It read, in part:

> While running for president of the United States, the former New York City Mayor Rudy Giuliani announced in a 2007 campaign advertisement, "I had prostate cancer, 5, 6 years ago. My chance of surviving prostate cancer—and thank God, I was cured of it—in the United States? Eighty-two percent. My chance of surviving prostate cancer in England? Only 44 percent under socialized medicine.
>
> To Giuliani this meant that he was lucky to be living in New York and not in York, England, because his chances of surviving prostate cancer seemed to be twice as high in New York. Yet despite this impressive difference in the five-year survival rate, the mortality rate was about the same in the United States and the United Kingdom.
>
> Why is an increase in survival from 44 percent to 82 percent not evidence that screening saves lives? For two reasons. The first is lead-time bias. Earlier detection implies that the time of diagnosis is earlier; this alone leads to higher survival at five years even when patients do not live any longer. The second is overdiagnosis. Screening detects abnormalities that meet the pathological definition of cancer but will never progress to cause symptoms or death (nonprogressive or slow-growing cancers). The higher the number of overdiagnosed patients, the higher the survival rate. In the United States a much larger proportion of men are screened by PSA testing than in the United Kingdom, contributing to the United States's higher survival rate.[35]

Gigerenzer explains that the higher survival rate in the United States, publicly advertised by Giuliani, is merely a statistical mirage. The earlier detection of prostate cancer due to routine PSA screening in the United States led to an exaggeratedly elevated survival rate, but the men did not live significantly longer than their counterparts in the United Kingdom. One poignant message was missing from Gigerenzer's paper: Not only did the US men not live longer than the UK men, they suffered immeasurably more unnecessary procedures and treatments because of routine PSA screening. Spearing sacred medical cows, like "early detection leads to cure," is fraught with peril.

By most accounts Rudy Giuliani was a very good mayor, perhaps even a great mayor. But his cleaning up of crime-ridden neighborhoods and his inspiring leadership on 9/11 does not make Rudy Giuliani an authority on prostate cancer. In that area he is just another celebrity unwittingly doing much more harm than good when it comes to men's health. Men believe that "America's Mayor" would never steer them wrong. That kind of power of influence needs to be handled with care.

In chapter 3 we heard from Professor Hal Arkes, PhD, who spent a good part of his career in Washington, DC, exploring health care trends. Arkes analyzed the two major trials, Göteborg included, that the US Preventive Services Task Force used to make its 2012 recommendation against routine PSA screening. Let me repeat his illustration of the reality of prostate cancer mortality: "Picture two auditoriums, each filled with a thousand men. One auditorium is filled with men who had PSA screening tests, and one auditorium is filled with men who had not been tested—8 men in each auditorium will die of prostate cancer. As hard as it is for some people to recognize, these two auditoriums represent the statistical reality of prostate cancer."[36]

Arkes's statistical prostate cancer metaphor might seem like a bitter pill to swallow, but it is better to build future strategies in prostate cancer detection and cure on clinical actuality, than to keep the truth obscured by unending statistical machinations and false hope.

There is another point in this discussion that needs attention. The National Cancer Institute has a yearly budget of about $5.1 billion.[37] Of that, only $288.3 million is allocated for prostate cancer research.[38] There is currently no cure for metastatic prostate cancer; we have a few ways to slow its growth, but the disease ultimately kills the man. Given that grim scenario, it is baffling that we spend more than $3 billion on PSA tests alone, when there is such an unmet financial need in finding improved methods of treating, if in fact not even a cure for prostate cancer.

WHO'S WATCHING THE WATCHERS?

On November 21, 1990, after having pleaded guilty to six counts of securities fraud, junk bond king Michael R. Milken was sentenced to ten years in federal prison.[39] (While Milken was in prison, a federal judge reduced his sentence, so he served only two years of the original sentence.) Here's an excerpt from comments by Judge Kimba M. Wood before imposing the original sentence:

> It has been argued that your violations were technical ones to be distinguished from accumulating profits through insider trading and that your conduct is not really criminal or that it is only barely criminal . . . these arguments fail to take into account the fact that you may have committed only subtle crimes not because you were not disposed to any criminal behavior but because you were willing to commit only crimes that were unlikely to be detected. We see often in this court individuals who would be unwilling to rob a bank, but who readily cash Social Security checks that are not theirs when checks come to them in the mail because they are not likely to be caught doing so. Your crimes show a pattern of skirting the law, stepping just over to the wrong side of the law in an apparent effort to get some of the benefits from violating the law without running a substantial risk of being caught.[40]

As the saying goes, Milken paid his debt to society, so why drag out this old matter of his being a felon, considering he is the founder of the Prostate Cancer Foundation, the nation's most prominent and wealthiest prostate advocacy group? First, Wood castigated Milken as one who would "commit only crimes that were unlikely to be detected." The sentiment of that line is woven into the fabric of this story, because many of the actors you've met have operated under those same auspices: promoting a screening test that does more harm than good is unlikely to be detected simply because there are so many tools at hand to obfuscate the truth.

Equally important is the financial connective tissue that reaches from advocacy organizations to industry and into the FDA. It's not criminal, but more like a disease of apathy and opportunism.

At least in this story, the FDA is a training ground for high-paid health care consultants whose FDA credentials make them ideal candidates for device and drug companies that need a former insider's help in the FDA approval process. For example, one prominent board member of Milken's foundation is former FDA Commissioner Andrew von Eschenbach, MD, who is also the president of Samaritan Health Initiatives, Inc., a health care policy consultancy that helps device makers negotiate their products through the FDA. It's a big bucks game and it is largely about having connections with the FDA.

On June 21, 2013, I e-mailed Frank E. Young, MD, PhD, who was FDA commissioner in 1986 when Hybritech's PSA test received its first approval for the management of men with prostate cancer. In my note I said:

A Freedom of Information Act–accessed transcript reveals a great deal of unease among the FDA advisory panel's decision to recommend approval. Their reluctance turned out to be prescient given that immediately following the 1986 FDA approval, the PSA test was marketed and used widely as an off-label screening tool, leading to countless men suffering needless radical prostatectomies. Was the agency not aware of this massive off-label use since many of the PSA screening promotions were highly public events, such as National Prostate Cancer Month?

Young (who was not personally accused of any wrongdoing) was forced to resign as FDA Commissioner in 1989, as the agency under his guidance was embroiled in several scandals; the most serious incident involved several FDA employees who pleaded guilty to accepting thousands of dollars from companies seeking approval for their generic drugs.[41] When asked about his departure from the FDA, Young commented, "Looking back is never a good idea."[42] I guess that philosophy was applied to my query about PSA. He never responded. Young has since moved on: he now serves on the boards of several pharmaceutical companies and is an adjunct partner in the health care venture capital firm, Essex Woodlands.[43]

As I mentioned previously, I also contacted Susan Alpert, MD, PhD, who was the director of the FDA's Office of Device Evaluation Center. She signed off on the 1994 approval of Hybritech's PSA test as an early detection/screening device. I posed a simple question about the PSA test approval:

> How could a test with a 78 percent false-positive rate be considered safe and effective? False positives produce many unnecessary surgeries so it does not, to my mind, meet the safety criterion. And a test that is wrong about 80 percent of the time certainly doesn't seem to fit the effectiveness criterion.

I never received a response from her either. Since leaving the FDA, Alpert has served on the board of several pharmaceutical companies and is currently a regulatory consultant for Accelmed, a firm that invests in medical-device companies—right up her alley.

David A. Kessler, MD, was FDA commissioner in 1994. During his tenure he became known for his attempt to have the agency regulate tobacco, which culminated in *FDA v. Brown & Williamson Tobacco Corp.* The Supreme Court ruled against the FDA. Kessler was also known for making the agency more vigilant in protecting consumers against unsafe products and inflated label claims. To his credit, he was the only official that responded to my queries. I asked Kessler via e-mail about the unease among members of the advisory panel as they debated Hybritech's application for approval of their PSA test a screening tool:

> Most disconcerting was William Catalona's presentation of trial data on behalf of Hybritech during which one alarmed panel member cited the 78% false-positive rate, saying that he had never seen a submission like this to the FDA. The worry was that putting an FDA stamp of approval on the test would place 30 million men each year in peril of having unnecessary treatments, such as life-changing radical prostatectomies. As we know, their worst fears came true. Did the FDA not realize the dangers involved in population screening of asymptomatic men?

Kessler replied on June 26, 2013:

> I am not sure I can help you. I have no recollection of being involved in the decision-making. This was all handled by [the Center for Devices and Radiological Health], no? Perhaps Bruce Burlington, who headed the Center, would know.

Remember, this was a decision involving 30 million to 40 million men. Even though he has no recollection of being involved in the PSA decision making, there is this quote attributed to him in a 1994 FDA press release following the PSA test's approval. It indicates that he was indeed engaged in the agency's role in this groundbreaking decision:

> This test (PSA)—used with other procedures—can help detect those men at risk for prostate cancer early on when more treatment options are available. . . . But for the test to help, men must be aware of the importance of early checkups and get them on a regular basis.[44]

The person Kessler suggested I contact, Bruce Burlington, MD, is listed on various enterprises as a "prominent independent consultant on pharmaceutical product development and regulatory affairs with more than 30 years of experience in regulatory affairs and drug development." Burlington was head of FDA's Center for Devices and Radiologic Health in 1994. After the tsunami of off-label use, Burlington sent out a series of warning letters to laboratories that were using PSA tests off label. The warning letters were largely ineffectual, as was the FDA's follow up.

Burlington never responded to my request to interview him.

I asked questions regarding the FDA approval process that warranted answers and, except for Kessler's brush-off, I was met with silence. You can judge for yourself, but from my research for this book, it has become apparent that FDA's relationship with industry and the revolving door that funnels ex-officials into lucrative positions with the device and drug makers has created a culture that looks the other way, far too often. The PSA test is evidence of that.

IN SEARCH OF THE HOLY GRAIL

Over the past several decades, we've seen a tremendous increase in the interest in prostate cancer, but unfortunately for the wrong reason: money.

The Holy Grail is said to be one of the vessels used by Christ during the Last Supper. It holds mystery and wonder to believers, and legend has it that some men have devoted their lives to searching for the spot where it is buried. I've used the Holy Grail metaphor in lectures as a way of demonstrating the ongoing search that I and others have conducted for a marker not that would not only identify prostate cancer, but would also enable us to separate the harmless slow-growing cancers from the fast-growing killers.

We need to go back to the drawing board and address three critical areas. *First,* we must gain better knowledge about how prostate cancer develops. Currently we do not understand this tumor's symbiotic relationship with the host and why at some unknown point in time a trigger goes off, setting the metastatic process in motion. My current research focuses on these challenges that need to be solved before true progress is made. *Second,* after we've identified a true cancer-specific marker, we need a treatment that works. This is where some of my thoughts on personalized medicine may offer clarity to this exciting new direction in cancer care.[45] Most promising is my earlier work in *cryoimmunotherapy,* which leads me to believe that our body's immune system offers a clue that will lead to a possible cure. But *third,* before we reach that point, the profit-over-patient culture needs to be looked squarely in the eye.

A well-respected colleague, Haakon Ragde, MD, an internationally renowned urologist and researcher from Norway, is currently working on a therapeutic approach toward strengthening the potential cryoimmunotherapic response by using the body's dendritic cells, which are vital components of the immune system. After seeing dramatic results in prostate cancer patients in the Philippines, he relocated his research to California. In a recent conversation, Ragde told me that he had achieved cures in patients with high-risk prostate cancer. But Ragde put a damper on my excitement over his results with his next remark.

> We had to close our clinical trial. Oncologists in the area referred us patients for the trial until they saw the good results. It scared the hell out of them to think that a simple and relatively inexpensive treatment—that works—might be under development. One guy confided in me that he loved the treatment, but he had three kids to put through college. We're packing up and moving the trial to Norway.[46]

Ragde is not paranoid. What he describes is the reality of Big Medicine. Despite incredible advances that have relieved the sick and suffering, the influence that money has on our health care system inspires deplorable stories like the one he tells. That said, the search for the Holy Grail continues and we will find it.

WHY NOW?

This book has been forming in my mind for almost two decades. I have told many of the issues and stories in it at lectures from Tucson to Tanzania to Fukuoka, and in long discussions that have, at times, challenged the patience of my colleagues, friends, and family—most notably my son, Michael, who all too often said, "You're not going to get the truth out by talking to us." Why have I waited so long to write a book about an issue that has consumed me for nearly half of my life? I actually began this book several years ago, but an internal voice urged me to wait for the right time—the right time being a point in my journey best suited to be heard and make a lasting impression, using truth as my ally.

Then one day in 2012, an associate remarked, "Dick, it amazes me that what you've been saying about PSA for decades is finally getting some traction. Why has it taken so long?" That's when it clicked. It had taken so long because no one voice was loud enough to break through the protective bubble around the PSA industry. More importantly, I realized that my 30-plus-year PSA war was not coming to an end. There was no white flag of surrender; it was a dangerous false détente of sorts that needed to be exposed. The bigger picture had not been told—one of greed and damaged men and government failure. That's why I waited, and why you are now reading this book.

Another reason I waited so long: In the movie *Backdraft,* Robert DeNiro's character, Donald "Shadow" Rimgale, is a fire department investigator specializing in arson. In one scene he relates his theory on fire: "It's a living thing, Brian. It breathes, it eats . . . the only way to beat it is to think like it. To know the mind of the fire, to know that this flame will spread this way across the door and up across the ceiling, not because of the physics of flammable liquids, but because it wants to."[47]

What I thought was a simple story of greed turned out to be a multilayered human drama. It took me a while to know the mind of the PSA tragedy and how it sparked and spread across the country and places beyond. Because to fully know the story, I also had to get to know the people involved in it.

In my research for this book, I've communicated with more than 60 people: laymen, physicians and scientists (listed in the Appendix), some of whom have been at loggerheads with my position on PSA screening. But every conversation was edifying in its own way and I always ended the discussion feeling better for having it. For instance, Fred Lee, MD, an innovator in his own right, who was there in the beginning of PSA screening, was adamant in his opinion and is respected for it.[48] Prostate cancer survivors Isaac J. Powell, MD, a noted prostate cancer specialist,[49] and well-known advocate Johnny Payne[50] both articulated the case for PSA screening among the underserved African American community.

Before I close, I want to leave you with a couple of takeaway messages that speak to the heart of this story. In the final days of writing this book, several papers on PSA screening and prostate cancer were published about the continuing exploitation of men and precious health care resources. One paper in particular illustrates the medical industry's defiance to reel in excessive use of costly technologies that have little to no proven benefit. During a 5-year period, there was a substantial increase in the use of highly expensive radiation therapy and robotic prostatectomies in men with low-risk prostate cancer who would most probably die of another cause.[51] I've discussed the terrible toll exacted on the bodies and minds of men because of the misuse of PSA, but it's also vital that I reinforce the economic toll to our system. Medical industry profiteers have squandered trillions of health care dollars since the PSA test was first brought to the market. Given the utter failure of PSA screening, scientifically and clinically, why are we continuing to drain our health care system by repeating something we already know does not work. The late Albert Einstein defined *insanity* as doing the same thing over and over again and expecting different results. Repeating the same mistakes borne at the beginning of the PSA saga borders on *criminal* insanity.

In the end, however, I have come away positive in my belief that honest robust dialogue is the only way to drive health care forward and expose the severe flaws in our system, beginning with the unholy alliances of medicine and industry. What ails biomedicine today requires an honest diagnosis. It is up to the president of the United

States to appoint FDA officials who live up to the trust society has placed in them.[52]

But the FDA, the nation's health-products gatekeeper, needs to answer the questions I pose in this book.

Succinctly stated by my colleague of 18-plus years, Mark R. Haythorn: "If PSA really was the biomarker deserving of FDA approval for detecting cancer in otherwise healthy men, there would be no need for debate, reanalysis and continued extensions of clinical trials."[53]

The agency owes an answer to millions of American men who underwent unnecessary procedures and surgeries that left many of them damaged for life. Remember the warning of Alexander Baumgarten, MD, PhD, one of FDA's own expert advisers: "Like Pontius Pilate, you cannot wash the guilt off your hands."[54]

IT'S 112 DEGREES IN TUCSON today, the day that I'm writing the final lines of this book. The hackneyed phrase "It's so hot you could fry an egg on the sidewalk" actually doesn't seem hackneyed at all as I cross the sunbaked parking lot to my office at the University of Arizona. The flag is at half-staff in honor of 19 fire fighters who perished battling a raging wildfire that seems to be consuming the whole state. It's almost hot enough here to make an old scientist pine for a laboratory in the northern city of Buffalo, New York.

I've watched football coaches in pregame locker room speeches tell their players to leave everything on the field. I appreciate the metaphor, imploring men to succeed at any and all costs to body and mind. But if you leave everything, there's nothing left for tomorrow's struggle. So for that reason, at least in theory, I won't leave everything on these pages—this is the end of my book, but not of my story.

—*Richard J. Ablin, PhD*
Tucson, Arizona, 2013

APPENDIX

A COMPILATION OF THE INDIVIDUALS CONTACTED IN THE COURSE OF THE WRITING OF THIS BOOK FOR THEIR OPINION ON PSA SCREENING FOR PROSTATE CANCER AND THE SEQUELAE THEREOF

In some instances interviews were conducted by Ronald Piana and in others by myself. These were combined for seamlessness.

1. **Abel, Paul D., MD,** Prof., Dept. Surgery & Cancer, Faculty of Medicine, Imperial College, London, UK. Prostate cancer authority—Abel believes PSA screening does more harm than good. June 2, 2013.
2. **Alpert, Susan, PhD, MD,** Director, FDA's Office of Device Evaluation in 1994, when the PSA test was approved as an early detection device. Did not reply to e-mail request for interview. June 12, 2013.
3. **Andriole, Gerald L., MD,** Robert Killian Royce Distinguished Prof., Dept. Surgery, Chief, Div. of Urologic Surgery, Washington Univ. School of Medicine, St. Louis, MO. Principal investigator of the PLCO PSA screening trial; concerned about overdiagnosis of prostate cancer due to PSA screening. January 11, 2013.
4. **Arkes, Hal R., PhD,** Prof., Dept. Psychology, Ohio State University, Columbus, OH. Authority in judgment of medical and economic decision making. March 12, 2013.
5. **Bahn, Duke K., MD,** Director, Prostate Institute of America, Ventura, CA. Prominent radiologist; early leading proponent of the use of color flow Doppler ultrasound, cryosurgery of the prostate and early collaborator with Fred Lee of relationship of PSA and prostate volume. July 12, 2013.
6. **Barry, Michael J., MD,** Medical Director, Stoeckle Center for Primary Care Innovation, Massachusetts General Hospital, Boston, MA; President, Informed Medical Decisions Foundation. Member AUA Guideline Panel, Early Detection of Prostate Cancer; editorialist on issues of PSA screening. December 31, 2012.

7. **Bennett, Charles L., MD, PhD, MPP,** CoEE Endowed Chair in Medication Safety and Efficacy, South Carolina College of Pharmacy and Univ. South Carolina, Columbia, SC. Uro-haemato-oncologist; prostate cancer survivor; prominent investigator of drug side effects; pro and con about PSA screening relative to how utilized. June 10, 2013.

8. **Bernstein, Harris, PhD,** Prof. Emeritus, Dept. Cellular & Molecular Medicine, Univ. Arizona, Tucson, AZ. Distinguished cell biologist and prostate cancer survivor. April 9, 2013.

9. **Boucher, Roland,** Invented (patented) first remote controlled toy car; expressed audacity of being required to take PSA test as requirement for pilot's license. February 4, 2013.

10. **Brett, Allan, MD,** Prof., Dept. Clinical Internal Medicine, Univ. South Carolina School of Medicine, Columbia, SC. Against PSA screening; co-author with Richard J. Ablin, *NEJM* article United States Preventive Services Task Force recommendation (Brett and Ablin, NEJM, 365, 1949, 2011). May 10, 2013.

11. **Bruskewitz, Reginald C., MD,** Prof. Surgery, Dept. Surgery and Urology, Univ. Wisconsin, Madison, WI. Voting member on the FDA 1993, Immunology Devices Panel Advisory Committee reviewing approval PSA screening. Did not reply to e-mail request for interview. January 4, 2013.

12. **Burlington, D. Bruce, MD,** Executive Vice President, Business Practices and Compliance, Wyeth Pharmaceuticals, Collegeville, PA. Independent consultant on pharmaceutical product development and regulatory affairs; wrote letter to the editor, "FDA Advises Labs Regarding Off-Label Use of PSA Assays" (*Burlington. Clin. Lab. News,* 21, 5, 1995). Did not reply to e-mail interview for request. June 21, 2013.

13. **Carter, Ballentine, H., MD,** Director, Adult Urology, Johns Hopkins School of Medicine, Baltimore, MD. Nationally and internationally highly regarded urologic surgeon; chair, AUA Guideline Panel, Early Detection of Prostate Cancer. June 3, 2013.

14. **Cavanagh, William A., MS,** VP R&D, IsoRay Medical, Richland, WA. Designer of clinical trials for cryoimmunotherapy and other therapies. June 26, 2013.

15. **Chou, Roger, MD,** Assoc. Prof., Div. General Internal Medicine, Dept. Medicine, Oregon Health & Science Univ., Portland, OR. Member of US Preventive Services Task Force recommending against PSA screening. January 16, 2013.

16. **Concato, John, MD, MPH,** Prof. Medicine, General Medicine, Director, Clinical Epidemiology Center, Yale Univ. School of Medicine; VA Connecticut Healthcare System, West Haven, CT. Screening, prognosis, and treatment strategies expert. Declined interview request, but offered to write post-publication commentary on the book. May 10, 2013.

17. **Cox, Alvin,** Prostate cancer survivor, educator and patient advocate who chose active surveillance over surgery; against PSA screening and unnecessary treatment of prostate cancer. October 4, 2012.

18. **Croswell, Jennifer, MD, MPH,** Medical Officer, Agency Healthcare Research and Quality. Member of US Preventive Services Task Force recommending against PSA screening. Did not reply to e-mail request for interview. December 18, 2012.

19. **Dahm, Philipp, MD, MHSc, FACS,** Prof. Urology, Univ. Florida, College of Medicine, Gainesville, FL. Coordinating editor, Cochrane Prostatic

Diseases & Urological Cancers Group; not in favor PSA screening. June 4, 2013.

20. **Dawley, Harold H., PhD,** Psychologist, former Director Psychology, VA Medical Center, New Orleans, LA. Prostate cancer survivor; against PSA screening and urological industry promoting unnecessary treatment of prostate cancer; authored book with Block: *Erectile Fitness Training for Good Sexual Health.* December 4, 2012.

21. **Ernstoff, Marc, MD,** Prof., Div. Hematology and Oncology, Dartmouth-Hitchcock Medical Center, Lebanon, NH. Consultant, FDA Immunology Devices Panel; for screening of cancer but not prostate. June 8, 2013.

22. **Gill, Lillian,** Senior Assoc. Director, Center for Devices and Radiological Health (CDRH), Department of Health & Human Services, Baltimore, MD. Signatory on 1998 FDA warning letter to Bayer Corporation for promoting off-label use of their PSA assay. Did not reply to e-mail request for interview. March 8, 2013.

23. **Glynn, Timothy, JD,** Prostate cancer survivor; principal attorney of qui tam action on PSA screening. December 28, 2012.

24. **Gold, Phil, MD, PhD, CC, OQ,** Prof., Dept. Medicine, McGill Univ. School of Medicine, Montreal, Quebec, Canada. Discovered carcino-embryonic antigen (CEA); opinion PSA screening does more harm than good. February 21, 2013.

25. **Greenspan, Michael B., MD,** Clin. Asst. Prof., Div. Urology, Dept. Surgery, McMaster Univ., Hamilton, Ontario, Canada. Specialist in erectile dysfunction; opinion PSA screening does more harm than good. April 3, 2013.

26. **Greenstein, Shane, PhD,** Elinor and Wendell Hobbs Professor, Management and Strategy at the Kellogg School of Management, Kellogg Chair, Information Technology, Northwestern University, Evanston, IL. Had serious post-prostate biopsy infection. Declined interview. January 30, 2013.

27. **Harris, Jules J., MD,** Clin. Prof., Div. Hematology-Oncology, Dept. Medicine, Univ. Arizona College of Medicine, Tucson, AZ. Member of 1993 FDA Immunology Devices Panel Advisory Committee reviewing approval PSA; not in favor of PSA screening. December 13, 2012.

28. **Haythorn, Mark R., MS,** Biomedical Information Search Specialist, Astra Zeneca, Wilmington, DE. Pro and con PSA screening relative to how used; longtime colleague RJA; co-author with RJA on PSA manuscripts. May 13, 2013.

29. **Hojnacki, Marie, PhD,** Dept. Political Science, Penn State Univ., University Park, PA. Advocacy and public policymaking; co-author of book *Lobbying and Policy Change.* Did not reply to e-mail request for interview. April 24, 2013

30. **Kemeny, Mary M., MD,** Chief, Dept. Surgical Pathology, North Shore Univ. Hospital, Manhasset, NY. Voting member of 1993 FDA Immunology Devices Panel Advisory Committee reviewing PSA test for screening. Did not reply to e-mail request for interview. January 4, 2013.

31. **Kessler, David, MD, JD,** Prof., Pediatrics, Epidemiology and Biostatistics, Univ. of California School of Medicine, San Francisco, CA. FDA Commissioner at the time of the approval of the PSA test for screening in 1994. "Had no recollection of being involved in the decision making." June 19, 2013.

32. **Ladoulis, Chas. T., MD,** Chairman, Telepathology Working Group at Department of Veterans Affairs, New York, NY. Chair, FDA Advisory Committee reviewing approval PSA test 1993. April 2, 2013.

33. **Lange, Paul H., MD,** Chairman Emeritus, Department of Urology, Univ. Washington, Pritt Family Endowed Chair in Prostate Cancer Research, Seattle, WA. Presenter on behalf of Hybritech at 1985 FDA Immunology Advisory Panel for the approval of PSA test as a prognostic marker for the recurrence of prostate cancer. Did not reply to e-mail request for interview. February 23, 2013.

34. **Lee, Fred, MD,** Prominent radiologist; early leading proponent of the use of color flow Doppler ultrasound; evaluation in collaboration with Duke Bahn on paradigm for distinguishing an increased level of PSA related to the volume of the prostate. June 27, 2013.

35. **Leflar, Robert B., JD, MPH,** Ben J. Altheimer Prof. Legal Advocacy, Univ. Arkansas for Medical Sciences, Little Rock, AR. 1985 FDA Immunology Advisory Panel for the approval of PSA test as a prognostic marker for the recurrence of prostate cancer and author of 1989 paper entitled "Public Accountability and Medical Device Regulation" (Leflar. 2 Harvard J.L. & Technology 1–84, 1989). April 16, 2013.

36. **Levitt, Joseph, JD,** Partner, Hogan Lovells, Washington, DC. In 1994, at the time of approval of the PSA test for the early detection of prostate cancer, served as FDA Deputy Director for Regulation Policy, Center for Devices and Radiological Health (CDRH). Did not reply to e-mail request for interview. January 4, 2013.

37. **Littrup, Peter, MD,** Director, Imaging Core and Radiological Research, Karmanos Cancer Institute, Wayne State Univ. School of Medicine, Detroit, MI. Was involved in early publications with Fred Lee, Gerald P. Murphy, et al. regarding the evaluation of PSA and its cost-effectiveness; proponent of cryosurgery and cryoimmunotherapy. June 14, 2013.

38. **McCormack, Robert T., PhD,** Head, Technology Innovation and Strategy, Veridex, LLC, Raritan, NY. Early scientist involved in development of PSA test at Hybritech. January 12, 2013.

39. **Markowitz, Harold, MD,** Head, Clinical Chemistry, Mayo Clinic, Rochester, MN. Chair 1985 and Member 1993 FDA Immunology Advisory Panels for approval of PSA test as a prognostic marker for the recurrence and early detection of prostate cancer; gave grave warning of consequences of population PSA screening. Deceased August 16, 2009.

40. **Mason, Malcolm D., MB,** Director, Institute Cancer & Genetics, Cardiff Univ. School of Medicine, Heath Park, Cardiff, UK. Prominent urooncologist, leader and member of several urology study groups in UK; opinion PSA screening does more harm than good. January 14, 2013.

41. **Moffat, Leslie E. F., MB, ChB,** Consultant Urologist, Dept. Urology, Univ. of Aberdeen, Aberdeen, Scotland. Opinion PSA screening does more harm than good (Moffat, *BJU Int'l*, 92, 340, 2003). March 22, 2013.

42. **O'Hara, Dennis,** 20-year prostate cancer survivor; nationally and internationally recognized educator and patient advocate; American Cancer Society Founder & Facilitator Man-to-Man prostate cancer survivor support program, Poughkeepsie, NY; author with Schwartz of book *Support Group*. December 6, 2012.

43. **Oppenheimer, Jonathan, MD,** CEO and Chief Pathologist (Uropathologist), OUR Labs, Nashville, TN. Early proponent that a term other than cancer be used for low-risk indolent cancers. March 16, 2013.

44. **Payne, Johnny,** Prostate cancer survivor; cancer community educator for several prostate cancer advocacy groups including "Us Too" and "Prostate Cancer Alliance"; pro PSA screening in patients with health care disparities. July 23, 2013.

45. **Polacheck, John W., MD,** Director of the Prostatitis Center, Tucson, AZ. International authority on male prostatitis. Did not reply to e-mail request for interview. May 20, 2013.

46. **Potosky, Arnold L., PhD,** Director, Health Services Research at Georgetown Univ., Lombardi Comprehensive Cancer Center, Washington, DC. Specialist in health services research and finance. Did not reply to e-mail request for interview. January 10, 2013.

47. **Powell, Isaac, MD,** Dept. Urology, Karmanos Cancer Institute, Wayne State Univ. School of Medicine, Detroit, MI. Involved with several prostate cancer advocacy groups particularly with the role of ethnicity and family history; pro PSA screening. May 22, 2013.

48. **Ragde, Haakon, MD,** Founder and Director, The Haakon Ragde Foundation for Advanced Cancer Studies, Seattle, WA. Authority of prostate cancer; early innovator of brachytherapy; proponent cryosurgery and cryoimmunotherapy innovations. July 1, 2013.

49. **Rittenhouse, Harry G., PhD,** Senior Director of Cancer Research at Gen-Probe Inc., San Diego, CA. Involved in contemporary and development of new generation PSA assays. Did not reply to e-mail request for interview.

50. **Robertson, Christopher, PhD, JD,** Currently Visiting Prof., Harvard Law School; Assoc. Prof., Rogers College of Law, Univ. Arizona, Tucson, AZ. Consulting attorney at private practice; specializes in bioethics and health policy, areas in which highly regarded. April 22, 2013.

51. **Sartor, Oliver, MD,** Piltz Prof. Cancer Research in Depts. Medicine and Urology, Tulane Univ. School of Medicine, New Orleans, LA. Uro-oncologist specializing in prostate cancer; pro-PSA as a means to risk-stratify patients; debated RJA "Should Men Get PSA Tests to Screen for Prostate Cancer?" *Wall Street Journal,* September 2012. March 21, 2013.

52. **Shapiro, Alan, MD,** Urologist in private practice, former Head of Urology, Cedars-Sinai Med. Center, Los Angeles, CA. Against PSA screening; President, Cure Prostate Cancer Now Foundation; principal figure with RJA in documentary *The Second Opinion.* June 20, 2013.

53. **Taube, Sheila E., PhD,** Consultant; retired scientist, NIH. Member 1993, FDA Immunology Devices Panel Advisory Committee reviewing approval PSA screening. December 12, 2012.

54. **Thompson, Ian M., MD,** Prof., Glenda and Gary Woods Distinguished Chair in Genitourinary Oncology, Univ. Texas Health Science Center, San Antonio, TX. Expert in prostate cancer. Declined e-mail request for interview. September 12, 2013.

55. **Valle, Ralph,** Prostate cancer survivor; nationally recognized community educator and early patient advocate; organized Us Too chapter, Phoenix, AZ. Declined e-mail request for interview. December 12, 2012.

56. **VanDevelder, Paul,** Screenwriter, journalist, author; prostate cancer advocate; against routine PSA screening and unnecessary treatment of prostate cancer. May 21, 2013.

57. **Vorstman, Bert, MD,** Surgeon, private practice, Florida Urological Associates, Coral Springs, FL. Author of *The Good, the Bad, and the Ugly of Prostate Cancer Treatment* and outspoken opponent of radical prostatectomy. May 7, 2013.

58. **Walter, Louise, MD,** Head, Div. of Geriatrics, Dept. Medicine, Univ. California and VA Medical Center, San Francisco, CA. Lead author, overuse of PSA in national Veterans Affairs health system. January 13, 2013.

59. **Welch, H. Gilbert, MD, MPH, PhD,** Prof., Medicine, The Dartmouth Institute, and Family and Community Medicine, Dartmouth Medical School, Hanover, NH. Antagonist of unnecessary PSA; author of *Overdiagnosed: Making People Sick in the Pursuit of Health.* March 6, 2013.

60. **Wilkes, Michael S., MD, MPH, PhD,** Prof., Medicine, Director of Global Health, Univ. of California Davis, Sacramento, CA. Early antagonist of PSA screening. February 19, 2013.

61. **Wilt, Timothy, MD, MPH,** Prof., Medicine and Core Investigator, Minneapolis VA Center for Chronic Disease Outcomes Research, Minneapolis VA Health Care System and the Univ. Minnesota School of Medicine, Minneapolis, MN. Principal investigator, Prostate Cancer Intervention versus Observation Trial (PIVOT) Study Group; member US Preventive Services Task Force recommending against PSA screening. June 14, 2013.

62. **Woolf, Steven, MD, MPH,** Director, Virginia Commonwealth University Center for Human Needs, Richmond, VI. Consults with government agencies and professional organizations on health policy, critical appraisal of evidence and matters related to preventive medicine; science advisor, US Preventive Services Task Force; 1985 FDA Immunology Advisory Panel for the approval of PSA test as a prognostic marker for the recurrence of prostate cancer. April 4, 2013.

63. **Yamey, Gavin, MD,** Lead of E2Pi, the Evidence-to-Policy Initiative at the UCSF Global Health Group; writer of medical policy. Did not reply to e-mail request for interview. December 11, 2012.

64. **Young, Frank, MD, PhD,** Senior Partner, The Cosmos Alliance, a Maryland Venture Capital firm. FDA Commissioner in 1986 when PSA test was first approved as prognostic marker for recurrence of prostate cancer. Did not reply to e-mail request for interview. June 18, 2013.

65. **Zietman, Anthony, MD,** Assoc. Director, Harvard Radiation Oncology Residency Program, Director, Genitourinary Service, Massachusetts General Hospital, Boston, MA. Past President, American Society for Radiation Oncology (ASTRO); member of AUA Guideline Panel, Early Detection of Prostate Cancer; vocal about overuse of expensive radiation treatments. April 17, 2013.

NOTES

INTRODUCTION

1. PSA levels are measured in nanograms per milliliter (ng/ml). Doctors use a specific level to determine whether to biopsy the patient's prostate gland for cancer. The "trigger" level for a biopsy has varied widely over the years. The current level for considering a biopsy is a PSA greater than 4.0 ng/ml. For the purpose of this story, I'll put John's PSA at 4.2 ng/ml.
2. H. Ballentine Carter et al., "Early Detection of Prostate Cancer: AUA Guideline," American Urological Association Education and Research, 2013, http://www.auanet.org/education/guidelines/prostate-cancer-detection.cfm.
3. Richard J. Ablin, "The Great Prostate Mistake," *New York Times,* March 10, 2010, http://www.nytimes.com/2010/03/10/opinion/10Ablin.html?pagewanted.
4. Richard. J. Ablin, et al., "Precipitating Antigens of the Normal Human Prostate," *J. Reprod. Fert.* 22 (1970): 573-574, and "Tissue- and Species-Specific Antigens of Normal Human Prostatic Tissue," *J. Immunol.* 104 (1970): 1329-1339.
5. The American Society of Clinical Oncology (ASCO) audited the 1995 study because serious scientific misconduct was found in a similar study that Bezwoda presented at ASCO's annual meeting in Atlanta.
6. M. Baker, "Common Test for Prostate Cancer Comes Under Fire. Urology Professor Who Once Championed the Procedure Now Calls It Virtually Useless," *Stanford Report,* September 22, 2004, http//news.stanford.edu/news/2004september22/med-prostate-922.html.
7. Multiple RAND studies, 1983–98. http://www.rand.org/health/feature/forty/health-services-utilization-study.htm.

CHAPTER 1: THE JUNGLE

1. The most common complication of chronic Chagas disease is a heart condition called chronic Chagas cardiopathy. Complications include enlarged heart, heart failure, severely altered heart rhythm, and heart attack.
2. Cryoablation is a clinical process that uses extreme cold (cryo) to destroy or damage tumor tissue (ablation).
3. Ward A. Soanes et al., "Remission of Metastatic Lesions Following Cryo-surgery in Prostatic Cancer: Immunologic Considerations," *J. Urol.* 104

(1970): 154-159; R. J. Ablin et al., "Prospects for Cryo-Immunotherapy in Cases of Metastasizing Carcinoma of the Prostate," *Cryobiology* 8 (1971): 271-279.

4. R. J. Ablin, "Cryoimmunotherapy," *Brit. Med. J.* 3 (1972): 476.

5. In immunology, an antigen is a substance that evokes the production of one or more antibodies.

6. Although still enigmatic, the controversial immune response I witnessed more than four decades ago (also called the abscopal effect [the word *abscopal* is derived from the Latin prefix *ab,* meaning *away from,* and the Greek word *skopos,* meaning *target*] is finally gaining attention in the medical literature. That experience, and others, persuaded me that there might be a single immune switch at the center of the hundred or so cancers that plague humankind. Our goal should be to find it. For further particulars see: W. Cavanagh, "The Abscopal Effect and the Prospect of Using Cancer against Itself," Prostate Cancer Research Institute, http://prostate-cancer. org/the-abscopal-effect-and-the-prospect-of-using-cancer-against-it.

7. After these striking immune responses to cryosurgery and the identification of PSA, I took a cursory look at the possible clinical relevance of PSA. For this purpose and by way of an example, I electrophoretically analyzed serum specimens from prostate cancer patients prior to and following treatment. I observed an elevated area based on the electrophoretic mobility of PSA in the pretreatment specimens, which was markedly reduced or absent related to treatment. And, in patients who had a clinical recurrence of disease, the previously reduced or absent area was increased. These observations, albeit preliminary, suggested that PSA could possibly be used following further studies for the prognosis of the recurrence of disease. I dropped this line of inquiry, which perhaps in hindsight was not the best choice given the subsequent FDA approval of the use of PSA as a "harbinger" for the recurrence of disease some 15 years later, as I wanted to continue my investigations for a possible prostate *cancer*-specific antigen.

8. Roswell Park Cancer Institute (RPCI), located in Buffalo, New York, became the first cancer center in the United States when it was founded in 1898 by Dr. Roswell Park. In 1974, RPCI received its National Cancer Institute (NCI) designation as a comprehensive cancer center. RPCI also serves as a member of the National Comprehensive Cancer Network (NCCN).

9. M.C. Wang et al., "Purification of a Human Prostate Specific Antigen," *Invest. Urol.* 17 (1979): 159-163.

10. For those with a further interest in the details of how my discovery of PSA in 1970 relates to the subsequent work of Chu et al., who comprised the Roswell Park team that purified the protein in 1979, the following critique may be noteworthy.

     The Roswell Park team was thoroughly familiar with my discovery of PSA in 1970. In 1973, Dr. Gerald P. Murphy, who was at the time director of the National Prostatic Cancer Project (NPCP) and of Roswell Park, invited me to submit a research grant application to the NPCP. I proposed to extend my recently published immunological studies of the prostate (Ablin et al. *J. Reprod. Fert.,* 22, 573, and *J. Immunol.,* 104, 1329, 1970 and Ablin, *Cancer,* 29, 1570, 1972) toward the "Immunochemical Grading of Primary and Metastatic Prostatic Tumors" (the title of the application). My application delineated various extraction and purification procedures. The grant was not approved.

Two of my published papers, dated 1970 and 1972, concerning the discovery of PSA were cited in the 1979 *Investigative Urology* article (the "1979 Article") co-authored by Murphy in which the Roswell Park team published the results of their work on PSA. Those same two papers of mine are referenced in US Patent 4446122, for "Purified human prostate antigen" (the "Patent") for which Chu et al. are listed as the inventors, primarily for the purposes of attempting to distinguish their work from mine. In essence, the Patent application contended that the PSA I discovered differs from the PSA that the Roswell Park team purified and patented. Others disagree; the disagreement turns on Roswell's interpretation of the two immunological methods utilized, precipitin and hemagglutination, and has recently been discussed in a communication in *The ASCO Post* (Richard J. Ablin, "Seeking Clarity on the PSA Story," 4, no. 13, August 15, 2013) as follows: "Hemagglutination studies . . . unequivocally demonstrated that PSA is present in human prostate extract, prostatic fluid, and seminal plasma. When viewed in context with precipitin data for the reaction between antisera to human prostate extract and prostatic fluid, a very strong reaction of identity—designating a commonality of the content of each—was obtained. This showed that PSA was present in human prostate extract and prostatic fluid. In concert with subsequent studies by Wang, et al. (*IRCS Med. Sci.*, 11, 327, 1983), it was shown that PSA in seminal plasma originated from prostatic fluid."

Patent Attorney Henry D. Coleman, PhD, JD, of Coleman & Sudol (New York, NY, presently Coleman Sudol Sapone PC, Bridgeport, CT) whom I retained, conducted a retrospective review of the claims made in the Chu et al. Patent. Dr. Coleman concluded that my "contribution to the art" (prior art) as reported in *J. Reprod. Fert.*, 22, 573, 1970 "anticipate[d] the claims set forth" in the Chu et al. Patent. A 2007 article speculated about the significance of the failure of the Patent application to cite my article in the *Journal of Reproduction and Fertility*: "Although citing this paper might or might not have altered the granting of the patent, perhaps with such evidence of previous work, the granting of the USA patent might be debatable." (Rao et al., *BJU Int'l.*, 101, 5, 2007). That said, the validity—or invalidity—of the patent is now a moot point; it expired May 1, 2001. I have never claimed, beyond the discovery of PSA, to have played a role in the development of the PSA test. However, as evidenced by several publications, Roswell Park has put forth a sustained effort to rewrite the history of my *discovery* of PSA. This approach has become an all-too-familiar feature of an unworthy effort to discredit my criticism of the disastrous public health policy of routine PSA screening. An abstract of a version of the subsequently published Rao article, cited above, which was presented at the 2005 Annual Meeting of the American Urological Association (May 21-26, San Antonio, TX, Abstract #892) unravel[ed] the controversy as follows:

> In 1970, Dr. Richard Ablin was the first to describe presence of precipitation antigens in the prostate . . . In 1979 Dr. Wang and his associates at Roswell Park described the isolation of a tissue-specific antigen from the prostate. . . . As they were the first to purify this protein they were credited for discovering PSA. . . . It is therefore misinterpreted in the literature that Wang et al. were the first to identify PSA in the human body taking the credit away from Dr. Richard Albin [*sic*] . . . . Although

the credit of purifying PSA goes to Dr. Wang, it was described 9 years earlier by Dr. Albin [*sic*].

In fact, several earlier publications, e.g., a 1999 article in the *Journal of Urology* put it even more succinctly: "Prostate-specific antigen was first identified in human prostate tissue extracts in 1970, purified and characterized in 1979, detected in serum in 1980," at which point the authors cited three references: Ablin et al: J. Reprod. Fert. 22:573, 1970; Wang, et al: Invest. Urol. 17:159, 1979; and Papsidero, et al: Cancer Res. 40:2428, 1980 (Polascik, et al. *J. Urol.*, 162, 293, 1999).

Subsequent to the foregoing, with the availability of resources, I was able to establish (unpublished data, December 1998) the molecular weight (one way to characterize the properties of a protein) of the PSA described in Ablin et al. (*J. Reprod. Fert.*, 22, 573, 1970) was 28-34 kD, commensurate with that established by Chu et al.

Enough said. I agree with the late Dr. Murphy on one point: "[W]e should not dwell on [when and by whom PSA was identified]. Rather, we should focus on the significance of the finding," and, if I might add, it's appropriate—and, far more often, inappropriate—use.

11. Purification is a series of processes that isolate a single type of protein from a complex mixture. Characterization is based on size, shape, and sequence concentration, and physiochemical properties.
12. *Milestones in Urology,* William P. Didusch Center for Urologic History, American Urological Association, Baltimore, 2005.
13. "The Man Behind the PSA Test," http://www.roswellpark.org/cancer/prostate/about/history-psa.
14. James Mohler, MD, and Donald L. Trump, MD, "Letter to the Editor: More Thoughts on PSA," and Richard J. Ablin, PhD, DSc (Hon), "Letter to the Editor: Dr. Ablin's Reply." Both letters appeared in *The ASCO Post* 13, 4 (September 15, 2012): 2, 82, 83.
15. Created in 1984, the US Preventive Services Task Force is an independent group of national experts in prevention and evidence-based medicine that works to improve the health of all Americans by making evidence-based recommendations about clinical preventive services such as screenings, counseling services, or preventive medications.
16. Shannon Brownlee and Jeanne Lenzer, "Can Cancer Ever Be Ignored?" *New York Times Magazine,* October 5, 2011.
17. Ibid.
18. Susan Sontag, *Illness as Metaphor and AIDS and Its Metaphors* (New York: Picador, 1977).

CHAPTER 2: A DECISION I THOUGHT I COULD LIVE WITH

1. M. C. Wang, et al., "Purification of a Human Prostate Specific Antigen (PSA)," *Invest. Urol.* 17 (1979): 159-163.
2. Lawrence D. Papsidero, et al., "A Prostate Antigen in Sera of Prostatic Cancer Patients," *Cancer Res.* 40 (1980): 2428-2432.
3. *Hybritech Incorporated v. Abbott Laboratories,* 849 F.2d 1446; 7 U.S.P.Q.2d 1191 Fed. Cir. 1988).
4. Organization for Economic Cooperation and Development, 2008.
5. Industry sponsorship and research outcome is discussed in *Cochrane Database of Systematic Reviews,* December 12, 2012.

6. Direct quotes or information from or about Howard Birndorf, Ivor Royston, and other members of the Hybritech experience are referenced from interviews conducted by historian Matthew Shindell, University of California, San Diego, or Mark Jones, PhD, UCSD. The interview transcripts are housed in the UCSD Library archives.

7. Thomas J. Perkins, "Kleiner Perkins, Venture Capital, and the Chairmanship of Genentech, 1976–1995," University of California, Berkeley, Regional Oral History Office, University of California, Bancroft Library, Berkeley, California Program in the University of California: "History of the Biological Sciences and Biotechnology," http://content.cdlib.org/view?docId=kt1p3010dc;NAAN=13030&doc.view=frames&chunk.id=div00001&toc.depth=1&toc.id=div00001&brand=calisphere.

8. Phil Gold, MD, PhD, author interview, March 18, 2013.

9. Mandeville Special Collections Library, University of California, San Diego, San Diego Technology History Project. Ivor Royston, PhD, Matthew Shindell, Historian, UCSD October 14, 2008, San Diego, California.

10. Perkins, "Kleiner Perkins."

11. Transcript, Immunology Devices Panel, 9:00 a.m. December 9, 1985, Room 703-727A, Hubert Humphrey Building, 200 Independence Avenue, SW, Washington, DC.

CHAPTER 3: WHAT THE *BLEEP* JUST HAPPENED?

1. Staging describes the severity of a person's cancer based on the extent of the original (primary) tumor and whether or not cancer has spread in the body. Contemporary practice is to assign a number from I to IV to a cancer, with I being an isolated cancer and IV being a cancer that has spread to the limit of what the assessment tool measures.

2. Laurence Roy Stains, "I Want My Prostate Back," *Men's Health,* January 28, 2010.

3. During active surveillance, a man is examined on a regular basis for signs of cancer progression using physical examination, the PSA test, and, sometimes, other tests such as CT scans, ultrasound, or MRI.

4. Jonathan Oppenheimer, MD, author interview, March 16, 2013.

5. Stains, "I Want My Prostate Back."

6. Ibid.

7. Gerald Andriole, et al, "Mortality Results from a Randomized Prostate-Cancer Screening Trial," *N Engl J Med* 360 (March 26, 2009): 1310-1319.

8. Zosia Chustecka, "Recommendation Against Routine PSA Screening in US," October 7, 2011, http://www.medscape.com/viewarticle/751159.

9. Mike Fillon, "Urology Meeting Highlights Prostate, Bladder Cancers," *Journal of the National Cancer Institute* (2012), doi: 10.1093/jnci/djs405.

10. Michael L. LeFevre, "Who?" interview in *The ASCO Post* 3, no. 10, July 1, 2012.

11. "New PSA Recommendations: The Debate over Prostate Cancer Screening Continues," *The ASCO Post* 3, 10 (July 1, 2012); see also "Urologists Outraged over Government Panel's Recommendation to Stop Life-Saving Prostate Cancer Testing," *PR Newswire,* May 21, 2012, http://www.prnewswire.com/news-releases/urologists-outraged-over-government-panels-recommendation-to-stop-life-saving-prostate-cancer-testing-152348925.html.

12. Michael Greenspan, MD, author interview, March 18, 2013.
13. LUGPA news release, May 21, 2012.
14. Gardiner Harris, "Panel's Advice on Prostate Test Sets up Battle," *New York Times*, October 7, 2011.
15. Quoted by Gina Kolata, "Prostate Test Found to Save Few Lives," *New York Times*, March 19, 2009.
16. Hal Arkes, PhD, author interview, March 15, 2013.
17. PIVOT Study Group, "Radical Prostatectomy versus Observation for Localized Prostate Cancer," *N Engl J Med* 367 (2012): 203-213.
18. Michael Barry, MD, author interview, December 31, 2012.
19. Richard J. Ablin, "The United States Preventive Services Task Force Recommendation against Prostate-Specific Antigen Screening—Point," February 7, 2012, doi:10.1158/1055-9965.EPI-12-0058.
20. Daniel DeNoon, "PSA Worthless for Prostate Cancer Screening? 'PSA Era Over,' Test's Pioneer Now Says," *WebMD Health News*, September 10, 2004, http://connecticare.com/GlobalFiles/HealthNews/article.asp?ID=091e9c5e8000eab3&Cat=0&Num=6.
21. Louise C. Walter, et al, "Prostate Cancer In Focus: Prostate-Specific Antigen (PSA) Screening in Older Men," *Journal of General Internal Medicine*, December 17, 2011.
22. "Prostate Cancer: Screening Guidelines," Memorial Sloan-Kettering Cancer Center, http://www.mskcc.org/cancer-care/adult/prostate/screening-guidelines-prostate.
23. Louise C. Walter, author interview, January 5, 2013.
24. T. Ming Chu, "Prostate Specific Antigen (PSA): The Historical Perspective," http://www.medicine.mcgill.ca/mjm/v02n02/psa.html.
25. Black men are at nearly double the risk of developing prostate cancer than their white counterparts. "Surveillance Epidemiology and End Results," www.cancer.gov, http://seer.cancer.gov/publications/ethnicity/prostate.pdf.
26. Streptococcal infections cause a variety of health issues, such as strep throat, scarlet fever, toxic shock syndrome, necrotizing fasciitis (flesh-eating disease), etc.
27. Slide presentation: Paul Lange, "PSA: Discovery and Uses," http://www.fhcrc.org/content/dam/public/events/IPCR/2_Lange_PSA_IPCR2012.pdf.
28. Transcript, "Immunology Devices Panel," 9:00 a.m., December 9, 1985, Room 703-727A, Hubert Humphrey Building, 200 Independence Avenue, SW, Washington, DC, page 31.
29. Gerald Murphy, MD, a pioneer in early prostate cancer research was a prominent figure in the development and promotion of the PSA test. Murphy was felled by a massive heart attack in 2000, while attending a conference in Tel Aviv.
30. Stamey et al., "Prostate-Specific Antigen as a Serum Marker for Adenocarcinoma of the Prostate," *N. Eng. J. Med.* 317 (1987): 909.
31. Ibid.
32. Oliver Sartor, MD, author interview, February 4, 2013.
33. Gina Kolata, "How Demand Surged for the Prostate Test," *New York Times*, September 29, 1993.
34. Ibid.
35. Direct quotes or information from and about Howard Birndorf, Ivor Royston, and other members of the Hybritech experience are referenced from interviews conducted by historian Matthew Shindell, University of

California, San Diego, or Mark Jones, PhD, UCSD. The interview transcripts are housed in the UCSD Library archives.

36. Ibid.

37. "A Guide For Success: Education and Best Practices Committee of NASPC 2010," http://www.naspcc.org/docs/NASPCC_GUIDE_EBPC_rev_4-11 .pdf.

38. Philips & Cohen LLP, "Representing Whistleblowers Across the Nation and Around the World," http://www.phillipsandcohen.com/News-Re ports-of-P-C-Cases/TAP-Pharmaceuticals-paid-875-million.shtml.

39. H. Gilbert Welch, MD, author interview, March 6, 2013.

40. Jeffrey McMurray, "Lawmakers Urging Prostate Cancer Screening," Yahoo News, January 14, 2005; http://votesmart.org/public-statement /105305/#.Uoz5C2SG1TM.

41. B. Schweitzer, "On the Cutting Edge," *Daily Freeman,* July 14, 2002, http://www.drcatalona.com/nationalmedia/dailyfreeman_kingston.htm.

42. Chris Woolston, "Many Men in 'Safe' PSA Range Have Cancer," Washington University in St. Louis: Archives, 1995-2003, http://wupa.wustl. edu/record_archive/1997/06-12-97/2457.html.

43. Gina Kolata, "It Was Medical Gospel, but It Wasn't True," *New York Times,* May 30, 2004, http://www.nytimes.com/2004/05/30/weekinre view/it-was-medical-gospel-but-it-wasn-t-true.html.

44. E. Johansson et al., "Long-Term Quality-of-Life After Radical Prostatectomy or Watchful Waiting: The Scandinavian Prostate Cancer Group Randomized Trial," *Lancet Oncology* 12 (2011): 891-899.

45. Kolata, "It Was Medical Gospel."

46. William J. Catalona, MD, "PSA Testing," slide show, https://docs.google .com/viewer?a=v&q=cache:OzRcpVErmUYJ:prostatenet.com/page/user files/ppt/12936917253—Catalona%2520PSA%25209-12-10.ppt+&hl=e n&gl=us&pid=bl&srcid=ADGEESh63SpM2MurI1nFJnLrLpO_iZxcB pPaqWx574pXPu_FNPOq06gnVdpSd5StkLlbx6eqoUhHJst66C_aog SO13kZtN47IEdJIh6zEMIgUFx_tLz01CbhfOpj7BuWT3gq4JcAGAhY &sig=AHIEtbTwDQmwwknCUUF0kRvkcU-X3m38kw.

47. All information and quotations are from Immunology Devices Panel Meeting transcript, June 29, 1993.

48. Marc D. Hauser, *Moral Minds: How Nature Designed Our Universal Sense of Right and Wrong* (New York: HarperCollins, 2007).

49. Jason Gale, "Surgery Restoring Penis After Prostate Surgery Increasing," Bloomberg.com, March 25 2013, http://www.bloomberg.com/news /2013-03-24/surgery-restoring-penis-after-prostate-cancer-increasing .html.

50. Jules J. Harris, MD, author interview, January 4, 2013.

51. William J. Catalona, "Two PSA Test Standards are Causing Problems in Screening For Prostate Cancer," http://www.drcatalona.com/quest/quest _spring09_5.htm.

52. "Best of the AUA Annual Meeting," Highlights From the 2010 American Urological Association Meeting, May 29–June 3, 2010, San Francisco, CA, http://www.ncbi.nlm.nih.gov/pmc/articles/PMC2931291/.

53. Jason Gale, "Prostate Exam Deaths From 'Superbug' Spur Inquiry Into Cancer Tests," Bloomberg.com, May 5, 2011, http://www.bloomberg .com/news/2011-05-05/prostate-exam-deaths-tied-to-superbug-ills-spur -cancer-test-inquiries.html.

54. Marcia Angell, "Industry-Sponsored Clinical Research: A Broken System," *JAMA* 300, 9 (2008): 1069-1071.
55. S. Loeb et al., "Complications After Prostate Biopsy: Data From SEER-Medicine," *J. Urol.* 186 (2011): 1830-1834.
56. F. Gilliland, W. Hunt, and C. Key, "Improving Survival for Patients with Prostate Cancer Diagnosed in the Prostate-Specific Antigen Era," *Urology* 48 (1996): 67-71.
57. Stuart Justman, "Uniformed Consent: Mass Screening for Prostate Cancer," *Bioethics* 26, 3 (2012): 143–48, 1467-8519, (online) doi:10.1111/j.1467-8519.2010.01826.x.
58. The prostate component of the PLCO (Prostate, Lung, Colorectal and Ovarian) Cancer Trial was undertaken to determine whether there was a reduction in prostate cancer mortality using PSA testing and DRE.
59. Malcolm Law Cited in: F.B. Charatan, "FDA Approves Test for Prostate Cancer," *Brit. Med. J.* 309 (1994): 628.2.
60. M. Kuriyama et al., "Multiple Marker Evaluation in Human Prostate Cancer With the Use of Tissue-Specific Antigens," *J. Natl. Cancer Inst.* 68 (1982): 99-105.

CHAPTER 4: THE COLOR OF MONEY

1. Inquirer Wire Services, "Gorbachev Says Arms Control Is Reason For Iceland Talks," *Inquirer* (Philadelphia), October 4, 1986, http://articles.philly.com/1986-10-04/news/26059500_1_arms-control-days-of-summit-talks-arms-race.
2. E. Ray Dorsey et al., "Funding of US Biomedical Research, 2003–2008," *JAMA* 303 (2010): 137, 142, citing Gail R. Wilensky, "Developing a Center for Comparative Effectiveness Information," *Health Aff.* 25 (2006): w572.
3. Congressional Budget Office, "The Overuse, Underuse, and Misuse of Health Care," http://www.cbo.gov/sites/default/files/cbofiles/ftpdocs/95xx/doc9567/07-17-health care testimony.pdf.
4. Dorsey et al, "Funding of US Biomedical Research."
5. Barton Moffatt and Carl Elliott, "Ghost Marketing: Pharmaceutical Companies and Ghostwritten Journal Articles," *Persp. Biology & Med.* 50 (2007): 18, 19, quoting a document that was produced in *Motus v. Pfizer,* 358 F.3d 659 (9th Cir. 2004).
6. Anthony Zietman, MD, author interview, January 14, 2013; all subsequent quotes from Zietman are from this interview unless indicated otherwise.
7. Peter Johnstone, et al. "Proton Facility Economics: The Importance of "Simple" Treatments," *Journal of the American College of Radiology* 9, no. 8 (August 2012): 560-563, http://www.jacr.org/article/S1546-1440(12)00170-6/abstract.
8. Ezekiel Emanuel and Steven Pearson: "It Costs More, but Is It Worth More?" *New York Times,* January 2, 2012, http://opinionator.blogs.nytimes.com/2012/01/02/it-costs-more-but-is-it-worth-more/.
9. Ibid.
10. James Yu, et al, "Proton Versus Intensity-Modulated Radiotherapy for Prostate Cancer: Patterns of Care and Early Toxicity," *Journal of the National Cancer Institute* 105, no. 10 (2013): 748, http://jnci.oxfordjournals.org/content/early/2012/12/13/jnci.djs463.abstract.

11. Intuitive Surgical Inc. (ISRG) IPO, http://www.nasdaq.com/markets/ipos /company/intuitive-surgical-inc-51057-2385.
12. Dan Carroll, "Should You Buy Stock in Intuitive Surgical After Its Earnings Hit?" *Motley Fool*, April 18, 2013, http://www.fool.com/investing /general/2013/04/18/intuitive-surgical-earnings-april-18th.aspx.
13. Timothy Wilson, MD, discusses prostate cancer screening options, http://www.cityofhope.org/prostate-cancer.
14. Advanced Urology Care P.C., http://www.urologicalcare.com/.
15. "Dealing With the Side Effects of Prostate Cancer Treatments," Cancer care.com, http://www.cancercare.org/connect_workshops/313-prostate _cancer_treatment_side_effects_2012-10-12.
16. Herb Greenberg: "Robotic Surgery: Growing Sales, but Growing Concerns," CNBC, March 19, 2013, http://www.cnbc.com/id/100564517.
17. Intuitive Surgical Quarterly Report Pursuant to Section 13 or 15(d) of the Securities Exchange Act of 1934, for the period ended June 30, 2013.
18. Lindsey Tanner, "'Da Vinci,' Robot Popular Among Surgeons, Has Regulators Worried About Safety," Associated Press, April 9, 2013.
19. Dennis O'Hara, author interview, December 6, 2012.
20. "CNN's Dr. Sanjay Gupta on da Vinci Surgery," YouTube, http://www .youtube.com/watch?v=vDjQXD3kc5A.
21. "Robotic Prostate Cancer Surgery Comes With Trade-off," NBCNews .com, October 13, 2009, http://www.nbcnews.com/id/33291388/ns/health -cancer/t/robotic-prostate-surgery-comes-trade-off/#.UXwV6Cu1RA.
22. Michael J. Barry, et al., "Adverse effects of robotic-assisted laparoscopic versus open retropubic radical prostatectomy among a nationwide random sample of Medicare-age men," *J. Clin. Onc.* 30, no. 5 (January 3, 2012): 513-518, doi: 10.1200/JCO.2011.36.8621.
23. Drs. Michael Barry and Floyd Fowler Jr., Informed Medical Decisions Foundation, http://informedmedicaldecisions.org/.
24. H. Ballentine Carter et al. "Early Detection of Prostate Cancer: AUA Guideline," American Urological Association Education and Research, 2013, http://www.auanet.org/education/guidelines/prostate-cancer-detec tion.cfm.
25. Robin Eisner, "FDA OKs First Robotic Surgical Device," http://abcnews .go.com/Health/story?id=118152&page=1.
26. Marc-Andre Gagnon and Joel Lexchin, "The Cost of Pushing Pills: A New Estimate of Pharmaceutical Promotion Expenditures in the United States," *PLoS Med.* 5 (2008): 29, 32 n.4. On p. 32 Gagnon and Lexchin discuss a PhRMA press release claiming that in the United States, the industry spent $29.6 billion on R&D in 2004 and $27.7 billion for all promotional activities, which the authors note excluded several major categories of promotional activities; they suggest that "pharmaceutical companies spend almost twice as much on promotion as they do on R&D." Whatever its precise size, such an enormous investment in promotional activities would be irrational if it did not change the behavior of physicians and consumers. Some such changes in behavior are of course salutary, if they drive a doctor away from an obsolete treatment and toward one that is instead effective, safe, and economical—one that just happens to be patented by a major pharmaceutical company.
27. Bruce Leff and Thomas E. Finucane, "Gizmo Idolatry," *JAMA* 299, no. 15 (2008):1830–32.

28. Joseph Mercola, "The Drugs Don't Work: A Modern Medical Scandal," Mercola.com, October 22, 2012, http://articles.mercola.com/sites/articles /archive/2012/10/22/modern-medical-scandal.aspx.

29. Richard Horton, "The Dawn of McScience," *New York Review of Books,* March 11, 2004, p. 9.

30. "'My Lobotomy': Howard Dully's Journey," NPR, November 16, 2005, http://www.npr.org/2005/11/16/5014080/my-lobotomy-howard-dullys -journey.

31. Ronald Kessler, *The Sins of the Father* (New York: Grand Central Publishing, 2012), 226.

32. "Walter Freeman's Lobotomies: Oral Histories," NPR, November 16, 2005, http://www.npr.org/templates/story/story.php?storyId=5014594.

33. Gina Kolata, "How Demand Surged for Prostate Test," *New York Times,* September 29, 1993, http://www.nytimes.com/1993/09/29/health/how -demand-surged-for-prostate-test.html?pagewanted=all&src=pm.

34. P. Bach, "Rising Costs of Cancer Care," *The ASCO Post,* August 15, 2011, 2, no. 12.

35. Ibid.

36. "PSA Standardization," Mayo Clinic, http://www.mayomedicallabo ratories.com/articles/hottopics/transcripts/2009/2009-10b-psa/10b-21 .html.

37. Dwight D. Eisenhower, "Military-Industrial Complex," Speech, Public Papers of the Presidents, Dwight D. Eisenhower, 1960, p. 1035–1040.

38. "Coach" Isreal Barken, MD, "High Intensity Focused Ultrasound-Focal Therapy: Lecture and Interview with Dr. Douglas Chinn," AskDrBarken .org, October 16, 2011, http://askdrbarken.org/site/high-intensity-focused -ultrasound-focal-therapy-lecture-and-interview-with-dr-douglas-chinn/.

39. "EDAP Partners With PanAm HIFU to Offer Ablatherm(R)-HIFU to Prostate Cancer Patients in Cancun, Mexico," *Globe Newswire,* March 15, 2012, http://globenewswire.com/news-release/2012/03/15/470915/249366/en /EDAP-Partners-With-PanAm-HIFU-to-Offer-Ablatherm-R-HIFU-to -Prostate-Cancer-Patients-in-Cancun-Mexico.html.

40. Douglas O. Chinn, "Prostate Cancer, To Screen or Not to Screen: What a Stupid Question or How the USPSTF Got It All Wrong," *Prostate Cancer Comm.* 29, no. 1 (2013): 5.

41. Burt Vorstman, author interview, December, 20, 2012.

42. Thomas King and Y. Zaki Almallah, "Post-Radical Urinary Incontinence: The Management of Concomitant Bladder Neck Contracture," *Adv. Urol.* (2012) :295798, doi: 10.1155/2012/295798, see also http://www.hindawi .com/journals/au/2012/295798.

43. "Manufacturer and User Facility Device Experience (MAUDE)," FDA, http://www.accessdata.fda.gov/scripts/cdrh/cfdocs/cfmaude/search.cfm.

44. Ibid.

45. Kimberly-Clark, http://www.kimberly-clark.com.

46. "The Depend Campaign to End Prostate Cancer" Brings Sports Legends Together to Celebrate National Prostate Cancer Awareness Month," *PR Newswire,* http://www.multivu.prnewswire.com/mnr/depend/39908.

47. Mark Cammarota, "Kimberly-Clark Launches Second Year of 'The Depend Campaign to End Prostate Cancer' With Expanded Roster of Sports Legends," June 3, 2010, http://investor.kimberly-clark.com/releasedetail .cfm?released=47631.

48. Andrew Adam Newman, "A Young Spin on Incontinence, in Spots Skirting Images of Aging," *New York Times*, March 28, 2012, http://www.nytimes.com/2012/03/29/business/media/depend-incontinence-products-take-a-youthful-turn.html.

49. M. Brunetti, et al., "Hypothalamus, Sexual Arousal and Psychosexual Identity in Human Males: A Functional Magnetic Resonance Imaging Study," *Eur J Neurosci*. 27, no. 11 (2008): 2922–27; doi: 10.1111/j.1460-9568.2008.06241.x.

50. Peter Loftus, "Pfizer Goes to Court to Protect Viagra," *Wall Street Journal*, June 13, 2011, http://online.wsj.com/news/articles/SB10001434052702304778304576377981860105532.

51. Camille Farhat, cited in Jason Gale, "Surgery Restoring Penis After Prostate Cancer Increasing," March 24, 2013, http://www.bloomberg.com/news/2013-03-24/surgery-restoring-penis-after-prostate-cancer-increasing.html.

52. Ibid.

53. "Manufacturer and User Facility Device Experience (MAUDE)," FDA, http://www.accessdata.fda.gov/scripts/cdrh/cfdocs/cfmaude/search.cfm.

54. Han Zhong, "Primer: The Medical Device Industry," American Action Forum, June 2012, http://americanactionforum.org/sites/default/files/OHC_MedDevIndPrimer.pdf.

55. True Diagnostics, Inc., http://www.truediag.com/press020513.html.

56. Jonathan Gornall, "Should YOU Have the New Test for Prostate Cancer? Flaws in the Usual Test Lead to Needless Ops that Can Wreck Sex Lives," *Daily Mail*, October 15, 2012, http://www.dailymail.co.uk/health/article-2218238/Prostate-cancer-Should-YOU-new-test-Flaws-usual-test-lead-needless-ops-wreck-sex-lives.html.

57. Malcolm Mason, MD, author interview, May 14, 2013.

58. Esther Napolitano, "On Cancer: News and Insights From Memorial Sloan-Kettering," Department of Surgery Chair Peter Scardino on Smarter Screening for Prostate Cancer, March 14, 2013.

59. Ibid.

60. John H. Ford, "Opko's 4KScore Could Generate Over $1.8 Billion Annually," October 3, 2012, http://seekingalpha.com/article/902221-opko-s-4kscore-could-generate-over-1-8-billion-annually.

61. "Forbes: Profile Phillip Frost," http://www.forbes.com/profile/phillip-frost/.

62. Investor's Hub, http://investorshub.advfn.com/boards/read.msg.aspx?message id=86325235.

63. Christopher T. Robinson, author interview, April 17, 2013.

64. Ben Goldacre, *Bad Pharma: How Drug Companies Mislead Doctors and Harm Patients* (London, UK: Faber & Faber, 2013).

65. Ibid.

66. OPKO, www.opko.com.

67. "OPKO Health Acquires Next Generation Prostate Cancer Tests," OPKO press release, January 23, 2012, http://investor.opko.com/releasedetail.cfm?ReleaseID=641539.

68. Andrew Pollack, "New Prostate Cancer Tests Could Reduce False Alarms," *New York Times*, March 26, 2013, http://www.nytimes.com/2013/03/27/business/new-prostate-cancer-tests-may-supplement-psa-testing.html?pagewanted=all&_r=0.

69. Richard Doll and Bradford Hill, "Lung Cancer and Other Causes of Death in Relation to Smoking," *Br. Med. J.* 2, no. 5001 (November 10, 1956): 1071–1081.

70. "A Frank Statement to Cigarette Smokers," ad in *New York Times,* January 4, 1954, http://www.tobacco.neu.edu/litigation/cases/supportdocs/frank _ad.htm.

71. K. D. Brownell and K. E. Warner, "The Perils of Ignoring History: Big Tobacco Played Dirty and Millions Died. How Similar Is Big Food?" *Milbank Quarterly* 87, no. 1 (March 2009): 259–294; doi: 10.1111/j.1468-0009.2009.00555.x; http://www3.nd.edu/~dhicks1/teaching/GFSP13/rea dings/13b-Brownell.pdf.

72. C. Everett Koop, "The Tobacco Scandal: Where's the Outrage?" National Press Club, 1998, http://tobaccocontrol.bmj.com/content/7/4/393.full.

73. Government Accounting Office, "Medicare Fraud, Waste, and Abuse: Challenges and Strategies for Preventing Improper Payments," GAO-10-844T, June 15, 2010, http://www.gao.gov/products/GAO-10-844T.

74. Ibid.

75. Radiotherapy Clinics of Georgia, http://www.rcog.com/what-we-do/pro state-cancer.

76. "Prostate Cancer Survival Rates: What They Mean," WebMD, http:// www.webmd.com/prostate-cancer/prostate-cancer-survival-rates-what -they-mean.

77. Radiotherapy Clinics of Georgia, http://www.rcog.com/what-we-do/pro state-cancer.

78. Ibid.

79. Gerald Chodak, MD, "Prostate Cancer Therapy Promoted Without Evidence?" *Medscape,* December 3, 2012, http://www.medscape.com/view article/775213.

80. Ibid.

81. "Georgia-Based Radiation Oncology Practice to Pay $3.8 Million to Settle False Claims Act Case," Department of Justice Office of Public Affairs, April 3, 2012, http://www.justice.gov/opa/pr/2012/April/12-civ-426 .html.

82. Charles Huggins et al. "Quantitative Studies of Prostatic Secretion," *J. Exp. Med.* 70 (1939): 543-556.

83. Marie L. Huber et al., "Interdisciplinary Critique of Sipuleucel-T as Immunotherapy in Castration-Resistant Prostate Cancer," *J. Nat'l. Cancer Inst.* 104 (2012): 273-279.

84. "Provenge TV Advertising Campaign Starts Next Month," CafePharma, http://www.cafepharma.com/boards/showthread.php?t=525190.

85. Jonathan S. Batchelor, "Provenge Wild Ride Blazes Trail for Immunotherapy," Cancer Network, December 6, 2010.

86. Transcript, US Food and Drug Administration, Center for Biologics Evaluation and Research, Cellular, Tissue and Gene Therapies Advisory Committee, March 29, 2007, http://www.fda.gov/ohrms/dockets/ac/07 /transcripts/2007-4291T1.pdf.

87. Ibid.

88. Luke Timmerman, "Dendreon CEO Mitch Gold Cashes Out With $26.7M Payday On FDA Approval," *Xconomy,* April 5, 2010 http:// www.xconomy.com/seattle/2010/05/03/dendreon-ceo-mitch-gold-cashes -out-with-17-5m-payday-on-fda-approval-news/.

89. Marilyn Chase, "Dendreon's Ups and Downs at FDA and on Nasdaq," *Wall Street Journal,* May 11, 2007, http://blogs.wsj.com/health/2007/05/11/dendreons-ups-and-downs-at-fda-and-on-nasdaq/.

90. "Michael Milken, 60,000 Deaths, and the Story of Dendreon," Deep Capture, September 15, 2009, http://www.deepcapture.com/tag/howard-scher/.

91. Paul Goldberg, "Dear FDA: Provenge Provokes Letters From Opponents, Advocates, Investors," *The Cancer Letter,* 33, no. 16 (April 27, 2007), http://www.deepcapture.com/wp-content/uploads/2009/07/CancerLetterMaha1.pdf.

92. Ed Silverman, "Provenge Activists Pressing Their Fight, Again," *Pharmalot,* August 4, 2008, http://www.pharmalive.com/provenge-activists-pressing-their-fight-again.

93. Katherine Hobson, "Dendreon Insiders Celebrate Provenge Approval With Stock Sales," *Wall Street Journal,* May 4, 2010, http://blogs.wsj.com/health/2010/05/04/dendreon-insiders-celebrate-provenge-approval-with-stock-sales/.

94. Ibid.

95. The term placebo is from the Latin "I shall please." Placebos are essentially a simulated or ineffectual medical treatment, such as an inert tablet. In the IMPACT trial, the placebo arm also received what is known as standard of care, in this case, chemotherapy plus the placebo.

96. Luke Timmerman, "Dendreon, With Key Milestone Now Reached, Sees Final Results on Immune-Boosting Drug Coming in April," *Xconomy,* January 14, 2009, http://www.xconomy.com/seattle/2009/01/15/with-key-milestone-now-reached-dendreons-final-results-on-immune-boosting-drug-due-in-april/.

97. Dan Longo, "New Therapies for Castration-Resistant Prostate Cancer," *N. Engl. J. Med.* 363 (2010): 479-481.

98. Goldberg, "Dear FDA."

99. Cecilia Lacks, PhD, "Provenge: The Latest Controversy," *Quest,* Summer 2012, http://www.drcatalona.com/quest/Summer2012/article5.html.

100. Sharon Begley, "Insight: New Doubts About Prostate-Cancer Vaccine Provenge," Reuters, March 30, 2012, http://www.reuters.com/article/2012/03/30/us-provenge-idUSBRE82T07420120330.

101. Ibid.

102. Ibid

103. Careers (Jobs), http://dendreonjobs.com/washington, accessed April 8, 2013.

104. Dendreon Corp. Securities Litigation, United States District Court for the Western District of Washington, Case Number 11-cv-01291-JLR, http://www.blbglaw.com/cases/00191.

CHAPTER 5: UNINTENDED CONSEQUENCES

1. "Anatomy of a Decision: Facts and Context in the "60 Minutes" Decision Not to Air a Tobacco Expose," from *Smoke in the Eye, Frontline* show #1413, air date April 2, 1996, http://www.pbs.org/wgbh/pages/frontline/smoke/cron.html.

2. Timothy B. Glynn, author interview, December 28, 2012. All subsequent quotes from Glynn are from this interview unless indicated otherwise.

3. Richard J. Ablin, PhD, on Behalf of the United States of America against 16 Named Pharmaceutical Companies—the Defendants, verified complaint filed August 21, 2003, US District Court, Eastern District of New York, No. CV 03-4287.

4. Ibid.

5. Leslie E. F. Moffat, "Pragmatism and PSA," *BJU International* 92 (2003): 340–341; doi: 10.1046/j.1464-410X.2003.04366.x.

6. Leonard S. Marks, "New Guidelines for PSA Testing Issued by American Urological Association (AUA)," 1st Quarter, February 22, 2000, http://www.usrf.org/news/2000PSAguidelines.html.

7. Tom Reynolds, "Experts Question Validity of PSA Testing for Life Insurance Policies," *Journal of the National Cancer Institute* 93, 13 (July 4, 2001): 968-970, http://jnci.oxfordjournals.org/content/93/13/968.full.

8. H. Ballentine Carter et al., "Early Detection of Prostate Cancer: AUA Guideline," American Urological Association Education and Research, Inc., 2013.

9. Scott Hensley, "Urologists Recommend Less PSA Testing for Prostate Cancer," NPR, May 3, 2013.

10. Ryan Jaslow, "Panel's PSA Test Recommendations Spark Debate Among Doctors, Cancer Survivors," CBS News, May 22, 2012, http://www.cbsnews.com/8301-504763_162-57439340-10391704/panels-psa-test-recommendations-spark-debate-among-doctors-cancer-survivors/.

11. Gina Kolata, "Prostate Test Found to Save Few Lives," *New York Times,* March 18, 2009, http://www.nytimes.com/2009/03/19/health/19cancer.html?_r=1&.

12. "Center: AUA Speaks Out Against USPSTF Recommendations," May 30, 2012, http://www.hisandherhealth.com/component/content/article/662-center-aua-speaks-out-against-uspstf-recommendations.

13. Kolata, "Prostate Test Found to Save Few Lives."

14. Thomas Stamey, "The Prostate Specific Antigen Era in the United States Is Over for Prostate Cancer: What Happened in the Last 20 Years?" *J Urol.* 172 (4 pt. 1) (October 2004):1297–1301.

15. "NFL and AUA Foundation Kick-off Fourth Season of Know Your Stats About Prostate Cancer," *PR Newswire,* September 11, 2012, http://www.prnewswire.com/news-releases/nfl-and-aua-foundation-kick-off-season-of-know-your-stats-about-prostate-cancer-169314296.html.

16. Paul Abel, MD, author interview, June 2, 2013.

17. Ibid.

18. Ibid.

19. E. David Crawford MD, "Prostate Cancer Awareness Week: September 22 to 28, 1997," *CA: A Cancer Journal for Clinicians,* December 31, 2008, http://onlinelibrary.wiley.com/doi/10.3322/canjclin.47.5.288/full.

20. Leon Jaroff, "The Man's Cancer: Prostate Cancer Is Reaching Epidemic Levels in the U.S.," *Time,* April 1, 1996, http://www.phoenix5.org/stories/famous/Schwarzkopf%20.html.

21. Jeffrey Krasner, "Schering-Plough Pleads Guilty to Conspiracy," *New York Times,* August 30, 2012, http://www.nytimes.com/2006/08/30/business/worldbusiness/30iht-drug.2639326.html.

22. Linda A. Johnson, "NJ Court Allows Whistleblower Suit Against Schering-Plough," Associated Press, May 25, 2007, http://legacy.utsandiego.com/news/business/20070525-1308-schering-ploughsued.html.

23. Steven Woolf, MD, Food and Drug Administration Center for Devices and Radiological Health Immunology Devices Panel, transcript, June 29, 1993.

24. Gardiner Harris, "Panel's Advice on Prostate Test Sets Up Battle," *New York Times,* October 7, 2011, http://www.nytimes.com/2011/10/08/health/policy/08prostate.html?_r=3&ref=todayspaper&.

25. Shannon Brownlee and Jeanne Lenzer, "Can Cancer Ever Be Ignored?," *New York Times,* October 5, 2011, http://www.nytimes.com/2011/10/09/magazine/can-cancer-ever-be-ignored.html?pagewanted=all.

26. Ibid.

27. Harris, "Panel's Advice on Prostate Test Sets Up Battle."

28. Ibid.

29. Transcript, Immunology Devices Panel, December 9, 1985, 100.

30. Transcript, Food and Drug Administration Center for Devices and Radiological Health Immunology Devices Panel, June 29, 1993.

31. Bruce D. Burlington, "FDA Advises Labs Regarding Off-label Use of PSA assays," *Clinical Laboratory News* 21, no. 5 (1995).

32. "PSA Test Off-Label Use for Diagnosis Addressed by FDA in Letter to Labs," *The Gray Sheet,* July 17, 1995, article #01210290008.

33. Ibid.

34. Ibid.

35. FDA Warning Letter from Lillian Gill, Director of Compliance Center Devices Radiological Health, FDA, to Helge H. Wehmeier, President/CEO of Bayer Corporation, August 25, 1998, http://www.fda.gov/downloads/ICECI/EnforcementActions/WarningLetters/1997/UCM066736.pdf.

36. Ibid. The lack of prostate cancer-specificity of the PSA test—a major concern expressed by some of the Panel Members of the 1993 Immunology Devices Advisory Committee for PSA screening—was becoming evident in the increasing number of unnecessary prostatic biopsies prompted by elevations of PSA that proved to be false positives, as no cancer was found. Therefore, "off-label" PSA tests—referred to as *PSA-related* concepts—were developed by several medical device companies in an effort to enhance PSA's ability to identify only patients with early prostate cancer and not those with other prostatic irregularities, such as prostatitis, that also elevate the PSA number. These PSA-related concepts include: free (f) PSA; %fPSA; total PSA and complexed PSA. For a detailed examination, please see a recent review: M. R. Haythorn and R. J. Ablin, "Prostate-Specific Antigen Testing Across the Spectrum of Prostate Cancer," *Biomarkers Med.* 5 (2011): 515. The PSA-related concepts, as explained have proved inadequate. Gill, PDA Warning Letter, August 25, 1998.

37. Gill, FDA Warning Letter, August 25, 1998.

38. Richard J. Ablin et al., "Precipitating Antigens of the Normal Human Prostate," *J. Reprod. Fert.* 22 (1970): 573-574, and "Tissue- and Species-Specific Antigens of Normal Human Prostatic Tissue," *J. Immunol.* 104 (1970): 1329-1339; R. J. Ablin. "Immunologic Studies of Normal, Benign and Malignant Human Prostatic Tissue," *Cancer* 29 (1972): 1570-1574.

39. M. Kuriyama et al., "Multiple Marker Evaluation in Human Prostate Cancer With the Use of Tissue-Specific Antigens," *J. Natl. Cancer Inst.* 68 (1982): 99-105.

40. Gill, FDA Warning Letter, August 25, 1998.

41. Reynolds, "Experts Question Validity of PSA Testing for Life Insurance Policies."
42. "Michael Wilkes, M.D., Ph.D," *i-One Health,* http://i-onehealth.org /michael-wilkes-m-d-ph-d/.
43. Dateline staff, "Provost to Take 'Appropriate Actions' in Academic Freedom Case," *UC Davis News and Information,* June 6, 2012, http://date line.ucdavis.edu/dl_detail.lasso?id=14072.
44. Ibid.
45. Michael Wilkes, "PSA Tests Can Cause More Harm than Good," *San Francisco Chronicle,* September 30, 2010, http://www.sfgate.com/opinion /openforum/article/PSA-tests-can-cause-more-harm-than-good-3172216.
46. Jonathan Eisen, "Report on 'Egregious Academic Freedom Violation' at #UCDavis," *The Tree of Life,* June 6, 2012, http://phylogenomics .blogspot.com/2012/06/report-on-egregious-academic-freedom.html #sthash.LD15uUII.dpuf.
47. Ibid.
48. Letter from Committee on Academic Freedom and Responsibility, Academic Senate, University of California, Davis, "Division Re: Egregious Academic Freedom Violation," May 18, 2012.
49. Letter from Robert Shibley, Senior Vice President, FIRE, to Linda P. B. Katehi, Chancellor, University of California, Davis, July 13, 2012.
50. Ibid.
51. Michael Wilkes, MD, PhD, author interview, February 27, 2012. All subsequent quotes are from this interview unless otherwise indicated.
52. Daniel Merenstein, "Winners and Losers," *JAMA* 291, no. 1 (2004): 15-16; doi:10.1001/jama.291.1.15, http://jama.jamanetwork.com/article.asp x?articleid=197947.
53. Ibid.
54. Ibid.

CHAPTER 6: THE HIDDEN TRUTH

1. "Mawé people," *Wikipedia,* http://en.wikipedia.org/wiki/Maw%C3%A9 _people.
2. "Virility," Oxford Dictionaries, http://oxforddictionaries.com/us/defini tion/american_english/virility.
3. Edith Hamilton, *Mythology: Timeless Tales of Gods and Heroes* (New York: Mentor Books, 1940).
4. "PSA Test Reduces Prostate Cancer Deaths by 40%," *PR Newswire,* March 11, 2012, http://www.bizjournals.com/prnewswire/press_releases /2010/03/11/DC69133.
5. Randi Londer Gould, "The General's Orders," *InTouch,* June 1999. (*InTouch* is no longer in publication.)
6. Ibid.
7. Ibid.
8. Richard J. Ablin, "PSA Assays," *Lancet Oncology* 1 (2000): 13.
9. Milan Zaviacic and Richard J. Ablin, "The Female Prostate and Prostate-Specific Antigen. Immunohistochemical Localization, Implications of this Prostate Marker in Women and Reasons for Using the Term "Prostate" in the Human Female," *Histol. Histopathol.* 15 (2000): 131-142.

10. *The Second Opinion,* directed by Sheri Sussmann (2008; Los Angeles: Eslconsulting, Inc., and Moxy Pictures).

11. Susan Brink, "PSA Test: Don't Do It, Say Angry Men," *Los Angeles Times,* August 4, 2008, http://latimesblogs.latimes.com/booster_shots/2008/08 /psa-test-dont-d.html.

12. Alan Shapiro, MD, author interview, January 22, 2013.

13. For example, see "Robotic Radical Prostatectomy Part I, Nerve Sparing," YouTube, http://www.youtube.com/watch?v=ugyHWDrPNZk.

14. Jean M. Mitchell, "Urologists' Self-Referral for Pathology of Biopsy Specimens Linked to Increased Use and Lower Prostate Cancer Detection," *Health Affairs* 31, no. 4 (2012): 741–74.

15. Government Accountability Office, "Report to Congressional Requesters, MEDICARE: Action Needed to Address Higher Use of Anatomic Pathology Services by Providers Who Self-Refer," June 2013, http://www.gao .gov/assets/660/655442.pdf.

16. Timothy Wilt, MD, MPH, author interview, June 20, 2012.

17. Alvin Cox, author interview, October 4, 2012.

18. Centers For Disease Control and Prevention Data Base, CDC Health Data Interactive, http://205.207.175.93/hdi/ReportFolders/ReportFolders.aspx ?IF_ActivePath=P,21.

CHAPTER 7: IT'S 112 DEGREES IN TUCSON

1. Eric Topol, *The Creative Destruction of Medicine: How the Digital Revolution Will Create Better Health Care* (New York: Basic Books, 2012).

2. Lewis Thomas, *The Medusa and the Snail: Medical Lessons from History* (New York: Penguin Books, 1979).

3. Ibid.

4. Richard J. Ablin, "The Great Prostate Mistake," *New York Times* March 10, 2010, http://www.nytimes.com/2010/03/10/opinion/10Ablin .html?pagewanted.

5. Prostate Conditions Education Council, www.prostateconditions.org.

6. E. David Crawford, quoted in "Prostate Conditions Education Council (PCEC) Comments on New AUA Clinical Guideline on Prostate Cancer Screening," *PRNewswire–US Newswire,* May 3, 2013.

7. Press release, "MDxHealth's ConfirmMDx(TM) Test Outperforms PSA in Prostate Cancer Detection Algorithm and Decision for Repeat Biopsy," MDxHealth, April 22, 2013, http://www.mdxhealth.com/news -and-events/press-releases-and-events?detail=1694495.

8. "E. David Crawford, MD: The Benefits of ConfirmMDx," YouTube, http://www.youtube.com/watch?v=XNyQHtkogig.

9. Ibid.

10. Ibid.

11. Jonathan Oppenheimer, author interview, March 16, 2012.

12. Robert Weiss, MD, commenting on an article by E. David Crawford, MD, "Rising PSA Level in a 46-Year-Old Man," *Oncology* 27, 5 (2013).

13. Francis Fukuyama, *The End of History and the Last Man* (New York: Free Press, 1992).

14. Sisshartha Mukherjee, *The Emperor of all Maladies,* (New York: Scribner, 2010).

15. Ibid.

16. Ibid.
17. Ibid.
18. Ibid.
19. Charles L. Bennett, personal communication, January 28, 2013.
20. Ibid.
21. Charles L. Bennett, author interview, March 12, 2013.
22. "Continence and Potency After Radical Prostatectomy," *Prostate Cancer UPDATE,* 5 (Winter 2000), http://urology.jhu.edu/newsletter/prostate_cancer53.php.
23. A. B. Brett and R. J. Ablin, "Prostate-Cancer Screening—What the U.S. Preventive Services Task Force Left Out," *N. Engl. J. Med.* 369 (2011): 1949.
24. Allan S. Brett, author interview, April 10, 2013.
25. "Lies, damned lies, and statistics," *Wikipedia,* http://en.wikipedia.org/wiki/Lies,_damned_lies,_and_statistics. The phrase itself is attributed to nineteenth-century British prime minister Benjamin Disraeli.
26. Jonas Hugosson et al., "Mortality Results from the Göteborg Randomized Population-Based Prostate-Cancer Screening Trial," *Lancet Oncology* 11 (2010): 725.
27. H. Schroeder et al., "Screening and Prostate-Cancer Mortality in a Randomized European Study," *N. Engl. J. Med.* 360 (2009): 1320.
28. H. Gilbert Welch et al., *Overdiagnosis: Making People Sick in the Pursuit of Health* (Boston: Beacon Press, 2011), chapter 4.
29. H. Gilbert Welch, "Making the Call," *JAMA* 306, no. 24 (2011): 2649-2650; doi:10.1001/jama.2011.1898.
30. Roger Chou, MD, MPH, author interview, January 16, 2013.
31. Roger Chou and Michael L. LeFevre, "Prostate Cancer Screening—The Evidence, the Recommendations, and the Clinical Implications," *JAMA* 306 (2011): 2721-2722.
32. H. Schroder, et al., "Prostate-Cancer Mortality at 11 Years of Follow-Up," *N. Engl. J. Med.* 366, no. 11 (March 15, 2012): 981-90; doi: 10.1056/NEJMoa1113135.
33. E. A. Heijnsdijk, et al, "Quality-of-life Effects of Prostate-Specific Antigen Screening," *N. Engl. J. Med.* 367, no. 7 (August 16, 2012): :595-605; doi: 10.1056/NEJMoa1201637.
34. Tara Parker-Pope, "New Data on Harms of Prostate Cancer Screening," *New York Times,* May 21, 2012, http://well.blogs.nytimes.com/2012/05/21/new-data-on-harms-of-prostate-cancer-testing/?hp&_r=1.
35. Gerd Gigerenzer and Odette Wegworth, "Five-Year Survival Rates Can Mislead," *BMJ* 346 (2013): f548.
36. Hal Arkes, PhD, author interview, March 15, 2013.
37. National Cancer Institute website, http:www.cancer.gov/aboutnci/Servingpeople/cancer-snapshots.
38. Ibid.
39. "The Milken Sentence; Excerpts From Judge Wood's Explanation of the Milken Sentencing," *New York Times,* November 22, 1990, http://www.nytimes.com/1990/11/22/business/milken-sentence-excerpts-judge-wood-s-explanation-milken-sentencing.html?pagewanted=all&src=pm.
40. Ibid.
41. Edmund L. Andrews, "A Scandal Raises Serious Questions at the F.D.A.," *New York Times,* August 13, 1989, http://www.nytimes.com

/1989/08/13/business/a-scandal-raises-serious-questions-at-the-fda.html
?pagewanted=all&src=pm.

42. Philip J. Hilts, "F.D.A. Commissioner Reassigned In Aftermath of
Agency Scandals," *New York Times,* November 14, 1989, http://www
.nytimes.com/1989/11/14/us/fda-commissioner-reassigned-in-aftermath
-of-agency-scandals.html.

43. Biography, Frank E. Young, MD, PhD, https://www.ewhv.com/team
/detail/frank_young.

44. "FDA Approves Test for Prostate Cancer," Federal Drug Administration
press release, August 29, 1994, quoted at http://scienceblog.com/commu
nity/older/archives/M/1/fda0245.htm.

45. Richard J. Ablin, "The Need for Personalized Therapy and Companion
Diagnostics in Prostate Cancer," *Biomarkers Med.* 5 (2011): 281-283.

46. Haakon Radge, author interview, July 1, 2013.

47. "Backdraft (film)," *Wikiquote,* http://en.wikiquote.org/wiki/Backdraft
_(film).

48. Fred Lee, MD, author interview, July 2, 2013.

49. Issac J. Powell, author interview, March 12, 2013.

50. Johnny Payne, author interview, January 28, 2103.

51. Bruce L. Jacobs, et al. "Use of Advanced Treatment Technologies Among
Men at Low Risk of Dying From Prostate Cancer," *JAMA* 309, no. 24
(2013):2587-2595; doi:10.1001/jama.2013.6882.

52. Modified from an astute comment by Marc Kirschner in his editorial, "A
Perverted View of 'Impact'," *Science* 340 (2013): 1265.

53. Mark R. Haythorn and Richard J. Ablin, "Prostate-Specific Antigen Testing Across the Spectrum of Prostate Cancer," *Biomarkers Med* 5 (2011):
515-526.

54. Transcript, "FDA: Center for Devices and Radiological Health Immunology Devices Panel," June 29, 1993.

INDEX